YOUR BODY DOES NOT HATE YOU, YOU'RE INFLAMED: BEAT THE BRAIN FOG, STOP THE BLOATING, AND CALM FLARE UPS

RICHARD M. PLANK

YOUR BODY DOES NOT HATE YOU, YOU'RE INFLAMED: BEAT THE BRAIN FOG, STOP THE BLOATING, AND CALM FLARE UPS

RICHARD M. PLANK

YOUR BODY DOES NOT HATE YOU, YOU'RE INFLAMED

CONTENTS

ONE

WHY EAT ANTI-INFLAMMATORY FOODS

Let's get one thing straight: if your body is constantly inflamed, it's not just a "symptom"—it's a slow burn sabotage. Inflammation is your immune system's way of dealing with stress, injury, toxins, poor diet, or even unrelenting mental pressure. Short-term? It's useful. Long-term? It's a wrecking ball for your health.

The Science Behind Inflammation and Disease

Inflammation isn't always the bad guy. It's your body's natural response to harm—like when you get a cut and it swells a bit. That's acute inflammation, and it helps you heal. But when the inflammation switch gets stuck in the "on" position, it turns chronic—and that's where the damage starts.

Chronic inflammation doesn't always scream for attention. It simmers quietly in the background, driving nearly every major lifestyle disease: heart disease, diabetes, autoimmune disorders, joint pain, skin flare-ups, gut issues, brain fog—you name it. The worst part? You can have it for years without knowing it.

It's like a fire inside your body. You won't always see the flames, but the damage is real.

Inflammatory Markers: What They Are and Why They Matter

Doctors don't guess when they talk about inflammation—they measure it. Certain blood markers tell the truth about what's going on under the hood. Here are a few of the big ones:

- CRP (C - reactive protein): One of the most common markers. If it's elevated, something is stirring the pot.

YOUR BODY DOES NOT HATE YOU, YOU'RE INFLAMED

- IL-6 (Interleukin-6) and TNF-alpha (Tumor Necrosis Factor-alpha): These are cytokines, proteins your immune system uses to communicate. High levels mean your body's in fight mode.
- ESR (Erythrocyte Sedimentation Rate): Another sign your body is dealing with inflammation—slower = better.

High levels of these markers aren't just numbers—they're red flags. They show up in people with chronic illness, and they tend to drop when people change their diet and lifestyle.

Research Highlights: Clinical Studies Supporting Dietary Intervention

Let's kill the myth that diet doesn't matter. It does. And there's proof.

- A 2015 study in the Journal of the American College of Cardiology showed that a Mediterranean-style, anti-inflammatory diet reduced the risk of heart disease and lowered CRP levels.
- In a 2018 randomized clinical trial, people with type 2 diabetes who followed an anti-inflammatory diet had improved blood sugar control and reduced insulin resistance.
- A 2021 review in Nutrients confirmed that anti-inflammatory foods—like fruits, vegetables, omega-3s, and whole grains—lowered IL-6 and TNF-alpha levels in people with autoimmune diseases and digestive disorders.
- Even mental health gets a boost. Multiple studies have linked anti-inflammatory eating patterns to reduced risk of depression, Alzheimer's, and age-related cognitive decline.

These aren't fringe ideas. This is well-documented science—and yet most people still reach for a pill before they look at their plate.

Common Inflammatory Conditions Improved by Diet

This isn't just about "feeling better." It's about taking back control. Here are the heavy hitters that respond well when you feed your body the right fuel:

- **Heart Disease and Hypertension.** Inflammation damages blood vessels. Over time, it leads to plaque buildup and stiff arteries—aka high blood pressure and heart disease. Anti-inflammatory foods (like leafy greens, berries, and omega-3s) can improve blood flow, lower blood pressure, and reduce CRP levels. Less inflammation, less heart risk. Period.

- **Type 2 Diabetes.** Chronic inflammation fuels insulin resistance—the root cause of type 2 diabetes. Sugar, processed carbs, and trans fats stoke the fire. Whole, anti-inflammatory foods help put it out. Studies show these diets help regulate blood sugar, improve insulin sensitivity, and even reduce medication dependency.

- **Autoimmune Conditions.** Autoimmune diseases like Hashimoto's, rheumatoid arthritis, lupus, and multiple sclerosis are rooted in an immune system gone haywire. Inflammation is the fire that keeps them burning. Cutting out inflammatory triggers—like gluten, dairy, seed oils, and processed foods—while loading up on nutrient-dense options can calm the immune response and reduce flare-ups.

- **Digestive Disorders (IBS, IBD, Crohn's, Colitis).** Your gut is ground zero for inflammation. What you eat either feeds the good bugs or fuels the bad ones. Processed foods? They wreck the gut lining. Anti-inflammatory foods? They help heal it. Many people with IBS, Crohn's, or colitis have seen massive improvements by eliminating inflammatory culprits (like gluten, dairy, or certain FODMAPs) and embracing gut-friendly choices like bone broth, leafy greens, and fermented foods.

- **Joint Pain and Arthritis.** Joint pain isn't just about wear and tear—it's often inflammation in disguise. People with arthritis often have elevated CRP and other inflammatory markers. Ditching sugar, fried foods, and refined carbs while adding omega-3s (hello, wild salmon and flaxseeds) and turmeric can help ease stiffness and swelling.

- **Skin Conditions (Psoriasis, Eczema).** Your skin is often a reflection of your gut and immune health. Psoriasis and eczema are linked to internal inflammation. Clean up the diet, reduce sugar, remove common triggers (like gluten and dairy), and you'll often see clearer skin within weeks. Not perfect—but significantly better.

- **Cognitive Decline and Neurological Health.** Brain fog, memory loss, and even serious conditions like Alzheimer's are all tied to—you guessed it—inflammation. Neuroinflammation affects how your brain functions. Anti-inflammatory diets (especially those rich in omega-3s, greens, berries, and olive oil) have been shown to support brain health and delay decline.

- **Chronic Fatigue and Fibromyalgia.** If you're constantly exhausted and your body hurts all over, inflammation could be at the core. Fibromyalgia and chronic fatigue often go hand-in-hand with high levels of inflammatory markers. While there's no one-size-fits-all fix, a clean, anti-inflammatory diet can dial down symptoms dramatically for many people.

Every bite you eat is either feeding the fire of inflammation or helping to put it out. You don't need to be perfect—but you do need to be intentional. Ditch the ultra-processed crap. Eat real food. Stick to stuff that actually grew, swam, walked, or flew. Watch how your body responds.

This isn't about trends. It's about taking your health back. Starting with your plate.
YOUR BODY DOES NOT HATE YOU, YOU'RE INFLAMED

WHO CAN BENEFIT FROM THIS DIET PLAN

Let's be clear: the anti-inflammatory diet isn't some niche trend or wellness fad for bored influencers. It's a practical, science-backed way to help your body function better—whether you're managing a diagnosed condition, dealing with mysterious symptoms doctors haven't figured out, or just want to stay out of the damn hospital in the first place.

This isn't just for the "sick." It's for anyone who's tired of feeling like crap and ready to take their health into their own hands.

1. People with Diagnosed Inflammatory Conditions

If your doctor has slapped a label on your symptoms—anything with the words "itis" or "autoimmune" in it—chances are inflammation is at the root of it. Conditions like:

* Rheumatoid arthritis
* Lupus
* Psoriasis
* Crohn's disease or ulcerative colitis
* Hashimoto's thyroiditis
* Asthma
* Type 2 diabetes
* Cardiovascular disease
* Chronic migraines

These aren't just names—they're signals that your immune system is in overdrive, mistaking your own tissues for the enemy. That means your body is literally inflamed from the inside out.

The anti-inflammatory diet helps calm that immune storm. It removes common dietary triggers and adds in foods that support healing and balance. Will it cure your condition? Probably not. But it can help dial down the flares, reduce your reliance on meds, and bring your quality of life back up.

2. People with a Family History of Inflammatory Diseases

Here's the cold, hard truth: your genes load the gun, but your lifestyle pulls the trigger.

If autoimmune diseases, heart issues, or diabetes run in your family, you're not doomed—but you are at higher risk. And the earlier you take action, the better.

Eating an anti-inflammatory diet before symptoms start is like investing in health insurance that actually works. It helps:

* Keep your immune system in check
* Regulate blood sugar and hormones
* Protect your gut (which is where your immune system lives)
* Lower your risk of inflammation-driven disease down the road

Don't wait for symptoms to smack you in the face. Prevention isn't sexy, but it's powerful—and way easier than dealing with a full-blown diagnosis.

3. Individuals Experiencing Unexplained Symptoms

If you've been told "everything looks normal" but you feel anything but normal, this part is for you.

Inflammation is a sneaky bastard. It can cause symptoms that don't fit neatly into a diagnosis—so doctors may miss it, or worse, brush you off. But your body knows something's off.

Here are some red-flag symptoms that inflammation might be the culprit:

* Persistent Fatigue: Not just "I didn't sleep well last night" tired. I'm talking "I woke up exhausted and feel like I'm dragging my body through wet cement" tired. Chronic fatigue is often driven by low-grade inflammation and hormonal imbalance.

* Brain Fog or Difficulty Concentrating: When your brain feels like it's moving through molasses, it's not just age or stress. Neuroinflammation (yes, your brain can get inflamed) messes with focus, memory, and mental clarity.

* Joint Pain or Stiffness: If your knees, hands, or back ache and you're not 90, that's your body waving a red flag. Especially if it comes and goes, or flares up after eating certain things.

* Digestive Issues: Bloating, gas, constipation, diarrhea, or alternating between all of the above? Inflammation messes with gut motility and microbiome balance. An anti-inflammatory diet can calm your gut down and help it function properly again.

* Unexplained Weight Changes: Inflammation messes with your hormones, insulin, and metabolism. Whether you're gaining weight for no reason or can't hold onto muscle, it might not be about willpower—it might be about chronic internal stress.

YOUR BODY DOES NOT HATE YOU, YOU'RE INFLAMED

- Sleep Disturbances: Waking up at 3 a.m. like your body's on high alert? Inflammatory foods can spike cortisol, mess with melatonin, and screw up your natural sleep rhythms.

- Mood Issues (Anxiety, Depression): This is a big one. Your gut and your brain talk to each other constantly. When inflammation messes with your gut, it can also tank your mood. Recent research even shows a link between systemic inflammation and depression.

If you're dealing with any of these symptoms and doctors can't give you answers—or you're tired of being told it's "just stress"—this diet could help you uncover what's really going on.

4. Athletes and Active Individuals Looking for Better Recovery

Even if you're in good shape, inflammation can still bite you. Every time you train hard, you're creating micro-damage in your muscles. That's part of how you get stronger—but if you don't recover properly, that low-level inflammation can pile up and slow you down.

Anti-inflammatory eating helps athletes:

* Recover faster
* Reduce muscle soreness
* Improve endurance
* Keep joints healthy
* Avoid overtraining burnout

We're not talking about gimmicky powders or "clean" processed bars. We're talking real food that helps your body repair itself and stay at peak performance without the crash.

5. Anyone Interested in Preventive Health

If you're not sick, not symptomatic, and just want to stay that way—congrats, you're already ahead of the game.

But here's the kicker: chronic inflammation builds up over time, often before symptoms show up. It's like a silent fire slowly weakening your system. Most people wait until they're diagnosed with something serious before making changes. Don't be like most people.

Eating anti-inflammatory foods isn't just about avoiding illness—it's about optimizing how you feel, think, move, and age. You'll have:

* More consistent energy
* Stronger immunity
* Better digestion

* Clearer skin
* Sharper focus
* Smoother moods
* Fewer "off" days

And you won't need to rely on coffee, energy drinks, or pharmaceuticals to keep your body running. That's the long game—and it pays off.

BOTTOM LINE: IF YOU HAVE A BODY, YOU'LL BENEFIT

INFLAMMATION AFFECTS EVERYONE. WHETHER IT'S OBVIOUS OR HIDING IN THE BACKGROUND, IT IMPACTS HOW YOU FEEL EVERY SINGLE DAY. YOU DON'T NEED TO WAIT FOR A DIAGNOSIS TO CLEAN UP YOUR DIET. IF YOU'RE BREATHING, YOU QUALIFY.

THIS PLAN ISN'T ABOUT RESTRICTION—IT'S ABOUT RECLAIMING CONTROL. IT'S ABOUT FUELING YOUR BODY WITH WHAT IT ACTUALLY NEEDS TO THRIVE, NOT JUST SURVIVE.

SO WHETHER YOU'RE MANAGING A CONDITION, CHASING ANSWERS, TRAINING HARD, OR SIMPLY AIMING TO LIVE BETTER FOR LONGER—THIS DIET ISN'T JUST FOR YOU.

IT'S ABOUT YOU.

WHY SOME FOODS WORK AGAINST YOU

You can eat all the kale in the world, but if you're still loading up on foods that trigger inflammation, you're basically trying to put out a fire while dumping gasoline on it. What you take out of your diet matters just as much—sometimes more—than what you put in.

Some foods work for your body. Others work against it. And once you understand why, you'll stop seeing food as just fuel and start seeing it as a choice that either supports healing—or sabotage.

How Foods Trigger Inflammation

Here's the quick and dirty science: when you eat inflammatory foods, your gut lining gets irritated, your blood sugar spikes, your immune system gets activated, and your body treats it like a threat. This kicks off what's called the inflammatory cascade—a domino effect of immune reactions, hormone imbalances, and cellular damage.

The end result? Swelling, pain, fatigue, brain fog, gut issues, skin flare-ups, and over time—chronic disease.

YOUR BODY DOES NOT HATE YOU, YOU'RE INFLAMED

Your body was built to handle occasional stress. But constant exposure to these inflammatory triggers keeps your system in panic mode. Over time, that takes a toll you feel.

Top Inflammatory Food Categories

Let's name names. These are the usual suspects—the foods that are most likely to keep your body stuck in the inflammation cycle:

1. Refined Carbohydrates and Added Sugars

These spike your blood sugar, fuel insulin resistance, and feed bad gut bacteria. Think:

* White bread
* Pasta
* Baked goods
* Sodas and sweetened drinks
* Candy, syrups, "low-fat" packaged foods (which are often sugar bombs)

They don't just give you a sugar rush—they light up inflammation markers like CRP and IL-6.

2. Industrial Seed Oils and Trans Fats

Canola, soybean, corn, cottonseed, sunflower—they're cheap, processed, and everywhere. These oils are high in omega-6 fats that throw your body's inflammation balance off.

Trans fats (partially hydrogenated oils) are even worse. They've been directly linked to heart disease and systemic inflammation. If it comes in a box or bag, check the label.

3. Conventional Dairy Products

Not everyone reacts to dairy, but for many people, it causes bloating, acne, congestion, or joint pain. The main culprits:

• Casein (a milk protein that can irritate the gut lining)
• Lactose (a sugar many adults can't digest properly)

Conventional dairy is also loaded with hormones and antibiotics, which can mess with your own systems. If you're sensitive, dairy can be a major inflammation trigger.

4. Processed Meats

These include:

* Deli meats
* Bacon
* Sausages
* Hot dogs
* Anything with "nitrates," "nitrites," or "smoke flavor"

They're full of preservatives, inflammatory fats, and compounds that have been linked to cancer and heart disease.

5. Artificial Additives, Colors, and Preservatives

If it has a color number (like Red 40 or Yellow 5), you probably shouldn't be eating it. These additives have been linked to hyperactivity, allergies, and immune dysfunction in sensitive people.

MSG, sodium benzoate, and other preservatives can also spark inflammatory responses in some individuals.

6. Alcohol

A little wine now and then might be fine. But chronic alcohol use disrupts gut health, taxes your liver, and causes systemic inflammation. It also screws with your sleep, your hormones, and your blood sugar.

Bottom line: moderation is key, and if you're actively trying to lower inflammation, cutting it out for a while can make a noticeable difference.

7. Gluten (for Sensitive Individuals)

Gluten isn't the devil for everyone—but for those with sensitivities, it can be a major inflammation bomb.

Celiac disease is the extreme. But even if you're not celiac, you could still have non-celiac gluten sensitivity that causes brain fog, joint pain, bloating, or skin issues.

If your body reacts poorly to gluten, cutting it out can be a game changer.

Food Sensitivities and Allergies

YOUR BODY DOES NOT HATE YOU, YOU'RE INFLAMED

Not all inflammation comes from obvious junk food. Sometimes it's from foods your body just doesn't like—even if they're "healthy" on paper.

Common Triggers

* Gluten
* Dairy
* Eggs
* Soy
* Corn
* Nuts
* Nightshades (like tomatoes, peppers, eggplant)
* Shellfish

Individual Variation

One person's superfood is another person's kryptonite. You could be eating clean, whole foods and still feel like crap—because your immune system sees something you eat every day as a threat.

Testing Options

- IgG/IgA food sensitivity tests: controversial, not 100% reliable, but sometimes helpful
- Skin prick or blood IgE allergy tests: more for true allergies than sensitivities
- Best option? An elimination diet—because your body doesn't lie.

Inflammatory Mechanisms in Specific Foods

Let's dig deeper into why certain compounds found in common foods mess with your body:

Advanced Glycation End Products (AGEs)

These form when food is cooked at high temperatures—like grilling, frying, or roasting. They promote oxidative stress and inflammation. Common sources:

* Charred meat
* Toasted bread
* Deep-fried anything

Use moist cooking methods (steaming, poaching, and slow-cooking) more often to reduce AGEs.

Lectins and Phytic Acid

Found in legumes, grains, and nightshades. These "anti-nutrients" can irritate the gut lining in sensitive individuals and block nutrient absorption. Most people tolerate them fine—but if you have autoimmune issues or gut problems, they might be worth limiting or preparing properly (soaking, sprouting, fermenting).

Omega-6 to Omega-3 Imbalance

Omega-6 fats aren't inherently bad—but we eat way too many of them (thanks to seed oils) and not enough omega-3s. This imbalance fuels chronic inflammation. You want to shift that ratio by reducing processed oils and eating more wild fatty fish, flax, chia, and walnuts.

Casein and Whey Protein Issues

Some people tolerate dairy proteins poorly—not just lactose. Casein (especially A1 casein from conventional cow's milk) can be pro-inflammatory. Even whey protein powders can cause issues if they're low quality or full of additives.

Nightshades and Their Effects

Tomatoes, peppers, potatoes, and eggplant contain alkaloids that can trigger joint pain or gut issues in sensitive people. Not everyone needs to avoid them—but if you have arthritis or autoimmune symptoms, it's worth testing.

Hidden Sources of Inflammatory Ingredients

Sometimes the worst offenders are hiding in "healthy" foods.

Check labels for:

* "Natural flavors" (which can mean almost anything)
* High-fructose corn syrup
* Carrageenan (found in some dairy-free milks and yogurts)
* Vegetable oils (soybean, canola, etc.)
* Maltodextrin
* Monosodium glutamate (MSG)
* Food dyes and preservatives

YOUR BODY DOES NOT HATE YOU, YOU'RE INFLAMED

If you can't pronounce it, or it sounds like it belongs in a chemistry lab—it's probably not helping you heal.

Decoding Food Labels to Identify Inflammatory Ingredients

Food companies are sneaky. They hide sugars under 50 different names (like "evaporated cane juice," "barley malt," "agave nectar"), and slap "heart healthy" on boxes full of inflammatory garbage.

Here's what to watch for:

* Long ingredient lists = red flag
* Oils other than olive, avocado, coconut = watch out
* Added sugar listed in the top 3 ingredients = skip it
* Anything with "artificial" or "natural flavors" = maybe (unless you trust the brand)

The fewer ingredients, the better. Whole foods don't need labels.

Bottom Line: Inflammatory Foods Aren't Worth the Cost

You can't out-supplement a crappy diet. And you can't fully heal if you keep eating the things that are causing the damage.

Cutting out inflammatory foods isn't about punishment—it's about power. You get to choose what goes in your body. And when you stop eating what's working against you, everything else becomes easier—your energy, your mood, your skin, your sleep, your focus.

This is where the real healing starts.

COOKING METHODS AND INFLAMMATION

You're doing the work. You're buying the right ingredients. But if you're nuking the life out of your veggies or charring your meat into a hockey puck, you're undoing a lot of the benefits.

Here's the truth most people don't hear: how you cook is just as important as what you cook.

Even the cleanest foods can become inflammatory depending on how you prepare them. Cooking methods can either preserve nutrients and lower inflammation—or trigger chemical reactions that stress your body out.

High-Heat Cooking & Inflammation: What You Need to Know

When you crank up the heat, things change—fast. Especially with protein-rich or fatty foods, high temperatures can trigger the formation of AGEs (Advanced Glycation End Products) and oxidized fats. These compounds are major drivers of inflammation, oxidative stress, and cellular aging.

You might not feel it immediately, but your cells do. And over time, it adds up—contributing to joint pain, cardiovascular disease, insulin resistance, and more.

How AGEs Form During Cooking

AGEs are toxic compounds that form when sugar reacts with proteins or fats during dry, high-heat cooking. This reaction is known as the Maillard Reaction—which makes food crispy, browned, and tasty... but also inflammatory.

Common AGE-rich foods include:

* Grilled or charred meats
* Deep-fried anything
* Roasted nuts or coffee at high temps
* Toasted bread
* Processed, browned, or dried snack foods (chips, crackers)

These compounds create oxidative stress in your body, disrupt healthy cell signaling, and promote chronic inflammation.

That doesn't mean everything needs to be boiled and bland. But it does mean you should rethink how often you're torching your food.

Problematic Cooking Methods

Let's break down the cooking methods that do your body more harm than good.

1. Deep Frying

Frying is a double-whammy:

* It usually uses refined seed oils (which are already inflammatory),
* Then heats them to extreme temperatures, oxidizing the fats.

YOUR BODY DOES NOT HATE YOU, YOU'RE INFLAMED

This creates free radicals, AGEs, and toxic byproducts. Even air-fried junk isn't a free pass if the ingredients or coatings are trash.

2. Grilling and Charring

Grilled meat smells amazing, but that crispy char? That's inflammation fuel.
High-temp grilling causes:

- AGEs in the meat
- PAHs (polycyclic aromatic hydrocarbons) from smoke and fat drippings
- HCAs (heterocyclic amines) from browned proteins

These are linked to cancer, gut irritation, and systemic inflammation. Occasional BBQ? Fine. Daily habit? Not ideal.

3. Dry Roasting at High Temps

Roasting nuts, seeds, or vegetables at high temps (400°F and up) oxidizes the fats and damages nutrients. You get better results—nutritionally and taste-wise—when roasting at lower temps with a bit of moisture.

4. Microwave Cooking Considerations

Microwaves aren't evil, but they can unevenly heat food, especially dense meals, leading to nutrient loss and overcooking certain areas. Use for reheating—not primary cooking—and avoid microwaving in plastic (more on that later).

Anti-Inflammatory Cooking Techniques

These cooking methods preserve nutrients, avoid AGEs, and actually enhance the anti-inflammatory power of your meals.

1. Water-Based Cooking

Steaming, poaching, boiling, braising—these methods use moisture, which prevents the formation of AGEs and keeps your food nutrient-dense.

- Steaming: Great for veggies—preserves texture and antioxidants.
- Poaching: Ideal for delicate proteins like eggs or fish.
- Braising: Low and slow—perfect for tougher cuts of meat or winter veggies.

2. Low-Temperature Cooking Methods

Cooking at or below 300°F helps prevent the breakdown of healthy fats and minimizes harmful compounds. Slow cookers and Dutch ovens are your best friends here. They make nutrient-dense, deeply flavorful meals with minimal effort.

3. Pressure Cooking Benefits

Pressure cookers (like Instant Pot) cook food quickly, retain nutrients, and reduce antinutrients like lectins and phytic acid—great for beans and grains.

It also destroys harmful bacteria without overcooking.

4. Raw Food Preparation

Some foods are most powerful in their raw state—full of enzymes, vitamins, and anti-inflammatory compounds.
Great raw options:

* Leafy greens
* Cucumbers, carrots, bell peppers
* Fermented raw foods (like sauerkraut)

But balance is key—too much raw food, especially for people with digestive issues, can be hard to tolerate.

5. Fermentation and Sprouting

These ancient methods unlock nutrients and improve digestion. They also boost your gut health—key to managing inflammation.

- Fermentation: Turns cabbage into sauerkraut, milk into yogurt, soybeans into miso. Adds probiotics and prebiotics.
- Sprouting: Reduces lectins and phytic acid in grains, legumes, and seeds, making them easier to digest and absorb.

Cooking Tools and Materials That Matter

Don't let your tools poison your food. Some cookware and containers leach harmful chemicals—especially under heat.

YOUR BODY DOES NOT HATE YOU, YOU'RE INFLAMED

Non-Toxic Cookware Options

- Cast iron: Durable, adds iron to your diet, great for searing at lower temps.
- Stainless steel: Non-reactive, safe, easy to clean.
- Ceramic-coated or 100% ceramic: Non-stick without toxic coatings.
- Glass bakeware: Inert and safe.
- Avoid: Teflon (especially old, scratched pans), aluminum (unless anodized), cheap nonstick pans.

Plastic vs. Glass Storage

Heat + plastic = chemical leaching. This includes BPA, phthalates, and other hormone-disrupting toxins.

- Store your food in glass (mason jars, Pyrex)
- Never microwave plastic containers
- Silicone is OK for cold use, but not great at high temps

Kitchen Tools That Support Anti-Inflammatory Cooking

- Steamer baskets
- Instant Pot or slow cooker
- Good blender or food processor for smoothies and soups
- Fermentation jars or crocks
- Sprouting jars or trays
- Sharp knives and cutting boards (you're more likely to prep real food if your tools don't suck)

Recipe Conversion: Making Comfort Foods Anti-Inflammatory

You don't have to give up your favorites—you just have to tweak them.

Example Swaps:

* White flour → almond, coconut, or cassava flour
* Vegetable oil → avocado, olive, or coconut oil
* Cow's milk → unsweetened almond, coconut, or oat milk
* Pasta → zucchini noodles, lentil or chickpea pasta
* Sugar → raw honey, date syrup, or just less sweetener overall
* Soy sauce → coconut aminos or tamari
* Breaded fried foods → air-fried or baked with nut flour coating

The key is flavor + function—make it taste good and feel good in your body.

Batch Cooking Strategies for Compliance

Life's busy. Cooking every single meal from scratch isn't realistic for most people. That's where batch cooking comes in.

Here's how to do it smart:

- **Pick 1 day a week (Sunday usually works) to cook multiple components**:

  * Roasted veggies (at a lower temp)
  * A couple proteins (slow-cooked chicken, salmon, boiled eggs)
  * Cooked grains or grain-free options (quinoa, cauliflower rice)
  * One pot of soup or stew
  * A sauce or dressing

- **Store in glass containers for mix-and-match meals throughout the week**

- **Freeze portions for emergency days**

- **Double recipes whenever possible—cook once, eat twice**

The more you prep ahead, the less tempted you'll be to order out or reach for crap when life gets hectic.

BOTTOM LINE: COOKING CAN HEAL OR HARM

FOOD IS MEDICINE—BUT IT CAN ALSO BE POISON DEPENDING ON HOW YOU COOK IT.

IF YOU'RE DOING ALL THE "RIGHT" THINGS BUT STILL FEELING STUCK, YOUR COOKING METHODS MIGHT BE PART OF THE PROBLEM. SHIFT AWAY FROM HIGH-HEAT, DRY, PROCESSED, PLASTIC-LACED HABITS—AND TOWARD SLOWER, LOWER, WATER-BASED, NUTRIENT-PRESERVING METHODS.

IT DOESN'T MEAN BORING. IT MEANS SMARTER. AND IT PAYS OFF IN ENERGY, CLARITY, FEWER FLARES, AND A STRONGER BODY—LONG TERM.

ANTI-INFLAMMATORY FOODS AND NUTRIENTS

YOUR BODY DOES NOT HATE YOU, YOU'RE INFLAMED

You can't out-supplement a bad diet. And you can't just remove inflammatory foods—you have to actively feed your body with the nutrients it needs to repair, restore, and regulate.

This section is your guide to building an anti-inflammatory plate—and doing it consistently.

The Anti-Inflammatory Food Pyramid

Think of this as your upgraded version of the outdated food pyramid that told you to load up on cereal and bread. This one actually supports your body's healing processes.

Here's what the anti-inflammatory food pyramid looks like (from base to top):

BASE – Every Day, Every Meal:

* Colorful veggies (especially leafy greens, cruciferous)
* Healthy fats (olive oil, avocado, nuts, seeds)
* Lean, clean proteins (fatty fish, pastured poultry, legumes)

MIDDLE – Daily or Several Times Weekly:

* Low-glycemic fruits (berries, apples, citrus)
* Whole, gluten-free grains (quinoa, buckwheat, oats)
* Fermented foods (sauerkraut, kimchi, kefir)
* Fresh herbs and spices (turmeric, ginger, garlic, rosemary)

TOP – Occasional Additions:

* Grass-fed red meat, eggs, organic dairy (if tolerated)
* Dark chocolate (min. 70% cacao)
* Red wine or green tea

Everything in this pyramid is designed to fight inflammation at the root—and provide steady, sustainable energy and resilience.

Superstar Anti-Inflammatory Foods

These aren't fads. These are the proven, evidence-backed heavy-hitters that should be showing up in your meals regularly.

1. Fatty Fish & Omega-3 Sources

* Wild salmon, sardines, mackerel, anchovies
* Plant-based: chia seeds, flaxseeds, walnuts (for ALA, less bioavailable)

Omega-3s help balance out inflammatory omega-6s and are critical for brain, heart, and joint health.
Tip: Aim for fish 2–3x a week, and consider a quality omega-3 supplement if you don't eat fish.

2. Leafy Greens & Cruciferous Vegetables

* Kale, spinach, Swiss chard, arugula
* Broccoli, cauliflower, Brussels sprouts, bok choy

These are packed with fiber, antioxidants, folate, and plant compounds that detoxify the body and reduce inflammatory markers.

3. Berries & Low-Glycemic Fruits

* Blueberries, raspberries, blackberries
* Apples, pears, cherries, citrus

High in polyphenols and flavonoids—plant antioxidants that protect cells from damage and regulate immune response.

4. Nuts & Seeds

* Almonds, walnuts, pumpkin seeds, sunflower seeds, chia, flax

Loaded with healthy fats, fiber, magnesium, and vitamin E. Keep portions moderate—about a handful a day.

5. Herbs & Spices

* Turmeric (curcumin): lowers NF-kB, a key inflammation trigger
* Ginger: reduces muscle pain, aids digestion
* Garlic: immune-modulating and antimicrobial
* Rosemary, cinnamon, oregano, cloves: high in polyphenols

Use them liberally. They're nature's pharmacy.

6. Olive Oil & Avocados
YOUR BODY DOES NOT HATE YOU, YOU'RE INFLAMED

* Extra virgin olive oil (cold-pressed) is a staple in Mediterranean diets for a reason.
* Avocados provide monounsaturated fats, fiber, potassium, and anti-inflammatory carotenoids.

7. Green Tea & Beneficial Beverages

* Green tea (EGCG), matcha, herbal teas like ginger and turmeric
* Bone broth (if tolerated): gut healing, joint-supporting collagen
* Filtered water: sounds basic, but dehydration = inflammation

8. Fermented Foods & Probiotic Sources

* Sauerkraut, kimchi, miso, kefir, and yogurt (if dairy tolerated)
* Kombucha (watch sugar content)

These feed your gut microbiome—which plays a massive role in systemic inflammation.

Key Anti-Inflammatory Nutrients and What They Do

Essential Fatty Acids (Omega-3s)

* Reduce inflammatory prostaglandins
* Support brain, heart, joint, and hormonal health

Antioxidants

* Fight oxidative stress and neutralize free radicals
* Found in colorful plant foods (vitamins A, C, E + polyphenols)

Polyphenols & Flavonoids

* Powerful plant compounds that reduce cytokine activity (inflammatory messengers)
* Found in tea, berries, dark chocolate, spices

Vitamins

* Vitamin A: Immune regulation, skin barrier repair (sweet potato, liver, leafy greens)
* Vitamin C: Collagen production, tissue repair, antioxidant (citrus, peppers, berries)
* Vitamin D: Immune modulation, bone health, anti-autoimmune (sunlight + supplements)
* Vitamin E: Protects cell membranes from oxidative stress (nuts, seeds, leafy greens)

Minerals

* Magnesium: Calms nerves, muscles, and inflammation (leafy greens, pumpkin seeds)
* Zinc: Immune support, wound healing (seeds, shellfish, legumes)
* Selenium: Antioxidant and thyroid support (Brazil nuts, seafood)

Fiber (Soluble + Insoluble)

* Soluble: Feeds gut bacteria, forms short-chain fatty acids (SCFAs) that lower inflammation
* Insoluble: Promotes regularity and detoxification
* Sources: legumes, veggies, fruits, flax, chia, oats

Phytonutrients: The Plant-Based Warriors

Plant-based compounds like sulforaphane (broccoli sprouts), quercetin (onions, apples), resveratrol (grapes, red wine), and anthocyanins (berries) modulate inflammatory pathways in the body.

They support detoxification, hormone balance, immune function, and even brain health.

Synergistic Food Combinations That Supercharge Benefits

Food isn't just a collection of nutrients. It's a synergy.

Here are some combos that amplify anti-inflammatory power:

* Turmeric + black pepper → dramatically boosts curcumin absorption
* Leafy greens + healthy fats (olive oil, avocado) → better absorption of fat-soluble vitamins
* Fermented foods + prebiotic fibers (onions, garlic, leeks) → nourishes your gut microbiome
* Green tea + citrus (lemon) → improves antioxidant stability

Eat these together. Let your food work harder for you.

Supplementation Guidelines

Supplements aren't a shortcut—but they can be a solid support when used smartly.

YOUR BODY DOES NOT HATE YOU, YOU'RE INFLAMED

When Supplements Make Sense:

* You're deficient (confirmed by lab work)
* You're dealing with high inflammation or autoimmune conditions
* You're not getting enough through food (e.g. Omega-3s, D3)
* You need therapeutic levels that food alone can't provide

Quality Considerations:

* Always choose third-party tested brands (like NSF, USP, and Informed Choice)
* Avoid fillers, dyes, unnecessary additives
* Choose bioavailable forms (e.g. methylated B vitamins, chelated minerals)

Dosage Guidelines (General, Not Personal Medical Advice):

* Omega-3s (EPA + DHA): 1,000–2,000 mg/day
* Vitamin D3: 2,000–5,000 IU/day (check blood levels)
* Magnesium (glycinate or citrate): 200–400 mg/day
* Curcumin (with piperine): 500–1,000 mg/day
* Zinc (gluconate or picolinate): 15–30 mg/day

Always check with a qualified practitioner, especially if you're on medications.

Interactions & Contraindications:

* Curcumin can thin the blood (watch if on anticoagulants)
* Too much zinc can deplete copper
* High-dose vitamin D needs adequate magnesium and K2 to balance calcium
* Supplements are powerful—treat them with respect

BOTTOM LINE: FOOD FIRST, SUPPLEMENTS SECOND

YOUR BODY IS CONSTANTLY RESPONDING TO WHAT YOU FEED IT. CHOOSE FOODS THAT REDUCE THE INTERNAL NOISE—NOT AMPLIFY IT.

LOAD YOUR PLATE WITH ANTI-INFLAMMATORY COLORS, TEXTURES, SPICES, AND FATS. EAT REAL FOOD, OFTEN. COOK IT WELL. SUPPLEMENT SMART WHEN NEEDED.

BECAUSE THE RIGHT FOODS DON'T JUST FEED YOU—THEY CHANGE YOU.

THE GUT CONNECTION

You can't talk about inflammation without talking about the gut. Period. If your gut is inflamed, you are inflamed—head to toe, inside and out. And in most people dealing with chronic symptoms or autoimmune flare-ups, gut dysfunction is a core piece of the puzzle.

Let's break this down and give you practical tools to actually do something about it.

Gut Microbiome's Role in Systemic Inflammation

Your gut is home to trillions of bacteria, fungi, and other microbes—collectively called the gut microbiome. These bugs aren't just freeloaders. They help digest food, produce nutrients, train your immune system, and even influence your mood.

But here's the deal:
When your gut microbiome is out of balance—a state called dysbiosis—your immune system gets triggered. Constantly. That low-grade, silent inflammation starts leaking into the rest of your body, affecting your brain, joints, skin, energy, and mood.

Key facts:

* 70–80% of your immune system lives in your gut.
* Your gut bacteria influence inflammatory cytokine production (like TNF-alpha and IL-6).
* Dysbiosis is linked to nearly every chronic inflammatory condition—from IBS to depression.

Intestinal Permeability ("Leaky Gut") Explained

Your gut lining is supposed to be selectively permeable—it absorbs nutrients and blocks harmful stuff. But when it gets damaged (from stress, processed foods, meds, alcohol, infections), it starts letting undigested food particles, toxins, and pathogens into your bloodstream.

That's leaky gut—and it's a major inflammation trigger.

Your immune system sees those invaders and launches an attack. Over time, this leads to chronic inflammation, autoimmune reactions, and symptoms that make no sense on paper (bloating, fatigue, rashes, joint pain, and brain fog).

Common causes of leaky gut:

* Processed foods (especially gluten, sugar, and industrial oils)

YOUR BODY DOES NOT HATE YOU, YOU'RE INFLAMED

* Alcohol and NSAIDs (like ibuprofen)
* Chronic stress
* Infections (like Candida or parasites)
* Antibiotic overuse

The Gut-Brain Axis and Neuroinflammation

Your gut and brain talk 24/7 through nerves (like the vagus nerve), chemical messengers, and immune signals. When your gut's inflamed, your brain knows it—and reacts.

This is the gut-brain axis in action.

Signs your brain is picking up on gut trouble:

* Brain fog
* Anxiety and panic attacks
* Depression
* Trouble focusing or remembering things
* Chronic headaches

Inflammatory signals from the gut can cross the blood-brain barrier and trigger neuroinflammation, which affects mood, cognition, and even neurological conditions like Alzheimer's and Parkinson's.

How to Heal the Gut Lining

If your gut lining is compromised, you need to stop the damage and give it what it needs to rebuild.

Step 1: Remove the offenders

* Cut inflammatory foods (sugar, gluten, processed junk, seed oils)
* Avoid alcohol and NSAIDs if possible
* Identify and treat infections (SIBO, Candida, parasites)

Step 2: Repair with nutrients

* L-glutamine – amino acid fuel for gut cells
* Zinc carnosine – supports mucosal healing
* Aloe vera, slippery elm, marshmallow root – soothing botanicals
* Collagen or bone broth – source of glycine and proline for tissue repair

Step 3: Rebuild the microbiome

(We'll get to that next)

Prebiotics, Probiotics, and Postbiotics

Let's clear the confusion.

Prebiotics – These are food for your good bacteria.

Sources:

* Garlic, onions, leeks, asparagus, Jerusalem artichokes, bananas, oats, flaxseeds

They feed beneficial bacteria like Bifidobacteria and Lactobacillus, which lower inflammation.

Probiotics – These are live beneficial bacteria you ingest.

Sources:

* Yogurt, kefir, sauerkraut, kimchi, miso, tempeh
* Supplements (choose high-quality, multi-strain)

Postbiotics – These are the byproducts of bacterial fermentation.

Things like butyrate, acetate, and propionate—they reduce gut inflammation and help heal the gut lining.

Short-chain fatty acids (SCFAs) are your gut's anti-inflammatory currency. You make them when you eat fiber and feed the right bugs.

Digestive Enzymes and Stomach Acid Balance

If food sits in your gut undigested, it ferments and feeds bad bacteria. That's where digestive enzymes and stomach acid come in.

Signs you're low in stomach acid (hypochlorhydria):

YOUR BODY DOES NOT HATE YOU, YOU'RE INFLAMED

* Bloating or fullness after meals
* Burping, gas, or reflux
* Undigested food in stool
* Nutrient deficiencies (B12, iron, magnesium)

Fix it:

* Drink apple cider vinegar or lemon water before meals
* Try bitters or betaine HCl (with practitioner guidance)
* Chew thoroughly and eat mindfully—digestion starts in your mouth

Digestive enzyme supplements can help break down proteins, carbs, and fats—especially during gut repair.

SIBO, SIFO, and Other Gut Disorders

When gut bacteria end up where they don't belong—like the small intestine—you get SIBO (Small Intestinal Bacterial Overgrowth). Same with SIFO (Fungal Overgrowth).

Symptoms:

* Bloating (especially after meals)
* Gas, cramping, diarrhea or constipation
* Food intolerances
* Brain fog and fatigue

These conditions often fly under the radar in conventional medicine but can be the root of ongoing inflammation.

Treatment often includes:

* Antimicrobial herbs (oregano oil, berberine, allicin)
* Gut-specific antibiotics (like rifaximin—if needed)
* Probiotics (strain-specific)
* Low-FODMAP diet (short term)

Testing Options for Gut Health

Testing is optional—but useful when your symptoms aren't improving or you want a clear picture.

Best options:

* Comprehensive stool test (like GI-MAP or Genova): detects pathogens, inflammation, enzyme levels, and more
* SIBO breath test**: checks for hydrogen or methane gas overgrowth
* Zonulin test: marker of leaky gut
* Organic acids test: looks at yeast, bacteria, and metabolic markers
* Food sensitivity panels (use with caution—elimination diets are often more reliable)

Always interpret these tests with a practitioner who knows what they're doing. A test without a plan is just expensive confusion.

The Elimination and Reintroduction Protocol

This is your go-to tool for identifying what's messing with your gut and inflammation levels.

Phase 1: Eliminate (3–6 weeks)

Cut the common triggers:

* Gluten
* Dairy
* Soy
* Corn
* Eggs
* Sugar
* Alcohol
* Caffeine
* Nightshades (if needed)

Focus on anti-inflammatory, gut-healing foods. Keep it clean.

Phase 2: Reintroduce (slowly, one at a time)

* Wait 3 days between each reintroduced food
* Track symptoms: energy, mood, skin, digestion, pain

If something triggers a reaction, remove it again and revisit it later.

This gives you direct, personal evidence of what your body does and doesn't tolerate.

YOUR BODY DOES NOT HATE YOU, YOU'RE INFLAMED

IF YOUR GUT IS A MESS, THE REST OF YOUR SYSTEM CAN'T RUN SMOOTHLY.
GUT HEALTH IS CENTRAL TO ENERGY, MOOD, IMMUNE FUNCTION, INFLAMMATION CONTROL, AND EVEN LONGEVITY.

REPAIR IT. FEED IT. SUPPORT IT.
YOU DON'T NEED TO BE PERFECT—BUT YOU DO NEED TO BE CONSISTENT.

THE GUT IS ALWAYS LISTENING TO YOUR CHOICES. WHAT ARE YOU TELLING IT TODAY?

LIFESTYLE FACTORS: YOUR LIFE AFFECTS YOUR INFLAMMATION, TOO

Food is powerful—but it's not the whole story.

You could be eating wild-caught salmon and organic kale all day, but if your sleep sucks, you're stressed to the edge, and your environment is full of toxins, you're still swimming upstream. Inflammation is not just about what's on your plate—it's also about what's going on in your *life*.

Here's where it gets real.

Stress Management Techniques

Chronic stress is one of the most powerful inflammation triggers. It activates the HPA axis, spikes cortisol, and over time, messes with blood sugar, immunity, digestion, and even your gut lining.

Here's how to break that loop:

- **Meditation and mindfulness**. Doesn't have to be fancy. Sit down, shut up, and breathe for 5–10 minutes. It rewires your nervous system. Use apps if it helps (Headspace, Insight Timer, etc.), or just sit in silence. It counts.

- **Breathing exercises**. Try box breathing: Inhale 4, hold 4, exhale 4, and hold 4. Or do extended exhales (inhale for 4, exhale for 8) to calm your system. Do it before meals, bed, or during stress spikes.

- **Yoga and gentle movement**. Not for the Instagram selfies—yoga calms the nervous system and supports lymphatic flow. Even just 10–15 minutes of gentle stretching can lower inflammation markers.

- Nature therapy. Forest bathing isn't just woo-woo. Research shows time in nature lowers cortisol and reduces pro-inflammatory cytokines. Walk barefoot. Sit in the sun. Watch the damn trees. It works.

Bottom line: Stress is inflammation. Manage it like your life depends on it—because it does.

Sleep Hygiene

If you're skimping on sleep, you're stoking inflammation. Period. Sleep is when your body heals, regulates hormones, and clears out inflammatory byproducts.

Here's how poor sleep hits you:

* Increases CRP (C-reactive protein), an inflammation marker
* Disrupts blood sugar and insulin sensitivity
* Amplifies stress hormone output
* Weakens gut barrier function and immune response

Create a sleep-friendly setup:

* Dark, cool, quiet room (aim for 60–67°F)
* No screens 60 minutes before bed (blue light = melatonin killer)
* Blackout curtains or a sleep mask
* White noise or earplugs if sound is an issue

Sleep-promoting habits:

* Go to bed and wake up around the same time every day
* Avoid caffeine after 2 p.m.
* Don't eat heavy meals right before bed
* Use magnesium (glycinate or threonate), CBD, or calming teas if needed

Common disruptors to fix:

* Sleep apnea (get tested if you snore or wake up groggy)
* Too much screen time
* Alcohol (wrecks REM sleep)
* Chronic pain or nighttime blood sugar crashes

YOUR BODY DOES NOT HATE YOU, YOU'RE INFLAMED

Physical Activity

Movement is anti-inflammatory medicine. But it's a Goldilocks zone—you need enough, but not too much.

How it helps:

* Improves circulation and lymph drainage
* Lowers visceral fat (a huge inflammation source)
* Boosts anti-inflammatory myokines from muscle activity
* Regulates insulin and cortisol

Best types of anti-inflammatory movement:

* Walking – underrated but massively beneficial
* Strength training – builds lean muscle and supports metabolic health
* Low-impact cardio – swimming, biking, elliptical
* Mobility and stretching – supports fascia and reduces stiffness
* Yoga, Pilates, tai chi – great for nervous system regulation

Intensity and duration tips:

* Aim for 150–300 minutes/week of moderate activity
* Don't overdo high-intensity stuff every day—your body needs recovery
* Mix strength and cardio for the biggest inflammation-lowering punch

Recovery strategies:

* Sleep, hydration, magnesium, rest days
* Gentle movement on off days (think yoga or walking)
* Listen to your body: soreness is fine—burnout and chronic fatigue are not

Overtraining red flags:

* Constant fatigue
* Injuries
* Cravings and poor sleep
* Low mood or irritability
* Declining performance

Environmental Factors

Your home, your products, your air, and even your wifi—they all influence your inflammatory load. And most of this stuff flies under the radar unless you're looking for it.

Toxin exposure in daily life:

* Plastics (BPA, phthalates)
* Pesticides (in food, lawns, bug sprays)
* Mold (especially hidden in bathrooms, basements, AC units)

Water quality concerns:

* Tap water often contains chlorine, fluoride, heavy metals, and drug residues
* Get a solid water filter (Berkey, Clearly Filtered, AquaTru—whatever fits your setup)

Air quality:

* Open windows often
* Use air purifiers (especially if you're in a polluted city or have pets)
* Avoid synthetic air fresheners and scented candles—they release VOCs

Household and personal care products:

* Ditch the toxic crap
* Choose natural or unscented cleaning and body care items
* Apps like Think Dirty or EWG's Skin Deep can help you choose safer stuff

EMF considerations:

* We don't have all the answers yet, but some people are more sensitive
* Use airplane mode while sleeping
* Don't keep your phone in your pocket 24/7
* Reduce exposure when you can—especially around sleep time

Social Connections and Community

YOUR BODY DOES NOT HATE YOU, YOU'RE INFLAMED

Loneliness and disconnection are inflammatory. Studies show people with poor social ties have higher CRP, cortisol, and risk of all-cause mortality.

Build your anti-inflammatory tribe:

* Prioritize real conversations, not just texts and social media
* Get involved in something bigger—volunteer, join a group, and be of service
* Connect regularly with people who uplift you (not drain you)

Human connection is healing. Make it part of your lifestyle medicine.

Time in Nature & Circadian Rhythm Alignment

You're wired to rise with the sun and wind down with the dark. Most of us are living like cave trolls—indoors, under artificial lights, out of rhythm.

Fix it:

* Get natural light in your eyes within 30 minutes of waking
* Go outside daily, even if it's just a short walk
* Dim lights and avoid screens after sunset
* Try camping or digital detox weekends to reset your rhythm

Mind-Body Techniques for Inflammation Reduction

This isn't just fluff—mind-body work rewires your stress response and brings your nervous system back into balance.

Options to explore:

* Somatic therapy
* Body scans and progressive relaxation
* Guided journaling
* Cold exposure (ice baths, cold showers)
* Acupuncture and massage

Pick what works for you. Don't force anything. If it makes you feel calmer and more connected, it's worth doing.

BOTTOM LINE: YOUR LIFE IS THE MEDICINE

EVERY CHOICE YOU MAKE—WHAT YOU EAT, HOW YOU MOVE, HOW YOU SLEEP, HOW YOU THINK, WHO YOU'RE AROUND—EITHER ADDS TO YOUR INFLAMMATION OR LOWERS IT.

YOU DON'T HAVE TO GET IT PERFECT. BUT YOU DO HAVE TO BE INTENTIONAL.

START WHERE YOU ARE. CLEAN UP WHAT YOU CAN. RECLAIM YOUR BODY FROM THE CHAOS. ONE SIMPLE HABIT AT A TIME.

MAINTENANCE AND LONG-TERM SUCCESS

Let's be real: anyone can go hard for a few weeks. But the real win? Making this way of living stick. This isn't a 30-day detox or a temporary reset. This is a foundational shift—a lifestyle that gets baked into your everyday routine without making you feel like a social outcast or a prisoner to your own kitchen.

Success long-term isn't about perfection. It's about consistency, adaptability, and staying grounded in your "why."

The 80/20 Approach to Sustainability

This isn't about being "on" or "off" the plan. That kind of thinking sets you up for burnout and guilt spirals. Instead, think 80/20.

* 80% of the time, you're dialed in: whole foods, anti-inflammatory staples, movement, sleep, boundaries, etc.
* 20% of the time, you loosen the reins a bit. Not a free-for-all, but a conscious decision to enjoy life without derailing your health.

Why it works:

* It gives you flexibility without falling off the wagon.
* It keeps the process mentally sustainable.
* It helps you build trust with yourself—you're in control, not the food.

This isn't a diet—it's a way of living. And life includes holidays, birthdays, vacations, and spontaneous nights out. The goal is to bounce back with zero drama.

Managing Setbacks and Flare-Ups

YOUR BODY DOES NOT HATE YOU, YOU'RE INFLAMED

Let's get one thing clear: flare-ups don't mean failure. They're data. Information. A signal from your body that something needs attention.

When you hit a bump, ask:

* Did I eat something I know doesn't sit well?
* Am I sleep-deprived?
* Under more stress than usual?
* Skipping movement or hydration?
* Feeling disconnected, isolated, or overwhelmed?

What to do next:

1. Don't panic – Inflammation is reversible.
2. Go back to your basics – Hydrate, eat clean, rest, and move gently.
3. Cut triggers temporarily – Eliminate known culprits for a few days to let your system reset.
4. Double down on gut support – Probiotics, bone broth, fermented foods, and simple meals.
5. Journal it – Get curious, not judgmental.

Healing is a messy, nonlinear process. Expect some waves. Just don't jump overboard every time you hit one.

Handling Social Pressure and Family Dynamics

You'll run into this—guaranteed. Not everyone will get it. Some will push back. Some will judge. Some will think you're being dramatic.

Here's how to navigate it without losing your mind:

Have a go-to explanation ready.

You don't owe anyone a medical breakdown, but a calm, firm line like:

* "This way of eating helps me feel better."
* "I'm managing inflammation and this works for me."
* "I've learned what fuels me and what flares me—and I'm choosing fuel."

Set boundaries without being a jerk.

You can be polite and still say no. Practice phrases like:

* "No thanks, that doesn't sit well with me."

* "I brought something I know works for me."
* "I appreciate the offer, but I'm good right now."

Lead by example, not lecture.

Let your results speak. When people see you with clearer skin, better energy, fewer symptoms—they'll start asking questions.

With family:

* Invite, don't impose. Cook delicious anti-inflammatory meals and let them enjoy it.
* Share resources only if they're open. (This book, for example.)
* Don't fight over food. Relationships come first. Be steady in your choices and let them adapt over time.

Creating New Food Traditions

Here's where it gets fun. You don't have to give up rituals—you just *remake them*.

Upgrade your traditions:

* Holiday meals? Make anti-inflammatory versions of classics.
* Comfort food? There's a way to make everything from lasagna to brownies without the inflammatory hit.
* Celebrations? Build new go-to meals and snacks you *look forward to*.

Cook with your people:

* Bring your partner or kids into the kitchen.
* Try new recipes together.
* Make food a connection point, not a battleground.

The goal isn't to feel deprived. It's to feel empowered and connected to your body—and to the people you love.

NOTE:

YOU'RE NOT CHASING QUICK FIXES ANYMORE. YOU'RE RECLAIMING YOUR HEALTH—ONE HABIT, ONE CHOICE, ONE DAY AT A TIME.

YOUR BODY DOES NOT HATE YOU, YOU'RE INFLAMED

Long-term success looks like:

* Knowing what works for you
* Trusting your body
* Bouncing back quickly
* Enjoying life without wrecking your health
* Feeling strong, clear, and energized more days than not

You don't need to be perfect. Just keep showing up.

This is how you win the war against inflammation—by living in a way that supports your body, not just once, but for good.

B
R
E
A
K
FAST

YOUR BODY DOES NOT HATE YOU, YOU'RE INFLAMED

Sweet Potato & Greens Hash

Prep Time: 10 minutes

Cook Time: 20 minutes

Servings: 2

2 medium sweet potatoes, peeled and diced small

2 tablespoons extra virgin olive oil

½ red onion, thinly sliced

1 red bell pepper, diced

2 cloves garlic, minced

2 cups chopped kale or spinach (destem kale if using)

½ teaspoon turmeric powder

¼ teaspoon freshly ground black pepper

Sea salt to taste

Optional toppings:

2 pasture-raised eggs (fried, poached, or soft-boiled)

½ avocado, sliced

1. Steam or boil the diced sweet potatoes for 5–7 minutes until just tender (this speeds up sauté time and keeps them from burning).

2. Heat 1 tbsp olive oil in a large skillet over medium heat. Add onions and bell pepper. Sauté for 4–5 minutes until soft.

3. Add another 1 tbsp olive oil to the pan and toss in the sweet potatoes. Cook for 6–8 minutes, stirring occasionally, until lightly crisp and golden.

4. Add garlic, turmeric, black pepper, and a pinch of sea salt. Stir well and cook for another minute until fragrant.

5. Add kale or spinach. Stir until wilted (about 1–2 minutes). Add a splash of water if the pan gets too dry.

6. Plate the hash. Top with fried or poached egg, or sliced avocado for a plant-based version.

Chia Pudding Power Bowl

Prep Time: 5 minutes

Soak Time: Overnight (or minimum 4 hours)

Servings: 2

½ cup chia seeds

2 cups unsweetened almond milk or coconut milk

½ teaspoon ground cinnamon

1 teaspoon pure vanilla extract (optional)

Pinch of sea salt

Toppings (per serving):

¼ cup fresh or frozen blueberries (wild if available)

2 tablespoons chopped walnuts

1 tablespoon unsweetened shredded coconut

1 teaspoon raw honey or date syrup

1 tablespoon hemp seeds

1. In a bowl or mason jar, combine chia seeds, almond/coconut milk, cinnamon, vanilla (if using), and a pinch of salt. Stir well to prevent clumping.

2. Cover and refrigerate overnight (or for at least 4 hours). Stir once after 10–15 minutes to redistribute the seeds

3. Divide the pudding into two bowls or jars. Top with blueberries, walnuts, shredded coconut, a light drizzle of honey or date syrup, and a sprinkle of hemp seeds.

4. Enjoy straight from the fridge, or let sit at room temperature for 10–15 minutes if you prefer it slightly warmer.

Green Smoothie with a Punch

Prep Time: 5 minutes

Servings: 1 large or 2 small

1 cup unsweetened almond milk (or coconut milk for creamier texture)

1 large handful of spinach or kale (destem if using kale)

½ frozen avocado (or ¼ fresh avocado + ice)

½ banana (ripe, for natural sweetness)

1 tablespoon ground flaxseed

1 scoop clean anti-inflammatory protein powder (pea, hemp, or grass-fed collagen—no added sugars or artificial junk)

½ teaspoon ground cinnamon

¼ teaspoon ground ginger (or ½ inch fresh ginger, peeled)

Optional: 1–2 ice cubes for extra chill, water for thinning

1. Add almond milk to the blender first. Then add greens, avocado, banana, flaxseed, protein powder, spices, and ice (if using).

2. Start on low, increase to high, and blend until smooth and creamy. Add a splash of water or more almond milk if it's too thick.

3. Pour into a glass or shaker bottle and sip slowly. For added gut support, drink it away from heavy meals.

Pro Tip:

If you're tight on time in the mornings, pre-pack smoothie bags (minus liquid and protein powder) and freeze. Just dump in the blender, add almond milk + scoop of protein, and go.

Turmeric Quinoa Porridge

Prep Time: 5 minutes

Cook Time: 15 minutes

Servings: 2

1 cup cooked quinoa (can be prepped ahead)

1 cup full-fat coconut milk (or light coconut milk for less richness)

½ teaspoon ground turmeric

¼ teaspoon ground cinnamon

¼ teaspoon ground cardamom

Pinch of sea salt

Optional: 1–2 teaspoons maple syrup or raw honey (added after cooking)

Toppings (per bowl):

2–3 chopped dates

1 tablespoon sliced almonds or crushed walnuts

½ apple or pear, thinly sliced

1 teaspoon tahini or almond butter (swirled in warm or dolloped on top)

1. In a small saucepan, combine cooked quinoa and coconut milk. Stir in turmeric, cinnamon, cardamom, and sea salt. Bring to a gentle simmer over medium heat.

2. Stir often, cooking for about 8–10 minutes, until the porridge thickens and the spices are well absorbed. Add a splash of water or more milk if it thickens too much.

3. Remove from heat and stir in honey or maple syrup if desired (skip if your toppings add enough sweetness).

4. Divide into bowls. Add chopped dates, sliced fruit, almonds, and a spoon of tahini or nut butter. Sprinkle with extra cinnamon if you like.

Make It Faster:

Cook a big batch of quinoa ahead of time and refrigerate or freeze in portions. You can have this porridge ready in under 10 minutes with zero stress.

Almond Flour Pancakes with Berry Compote

Prep Time: 10 minutes

Cook Time: 15 minutes

Servings: 2 (makes about 6 small pancakes)

Pancake Ingredients:

1 cup almond flour

2 large pasture-raised eggs

¼ teaspoon baking soda

¼ cup unsweetened almond or coconut milk

1 teaspoon vanilla extract (optional)

Pinch of sea salt

Avocado oil (for pan)

Berry Compote Ingredients:

1 cup frozen or fresh blueberries

½ cup raspberries (fresh or frozen)

Zest of ½ lemon

1–2 teaspoons fresh lemon juice

Optional: 1–2 teaspoons raw honey or date syrup (only if needed)

Make the Pancakes:

1. In a bowl, whisk together eggs, almond milk, and vanilla. Add almond flour, baking soda, and salt. Stir to form a smooth batter—thick but pourable. Let it sit for 2–3 minutes to thicken slightly.

2. Heat a nonstick skillet or griddle over medium heat and brush lightly with avocado oil. Pour batter into small rounds (about 2–3 inches wide).

3. Cook for 2–3 minutes on one side until bubbles form and the edges firm up. Flip and cook another 1–2 minutes. Keep warm while you finish the rest.

Make the Berry Compote:

4. In a small saucepan over medium heat, add blueberries, raspberries, lemon zest, and juice. Stir occasionally and simmer for 5–7 minutes until berries break down into a syrupy compote. Sweeten only if needed.

Serve: Stack pancakes on plates, spoon warm berry compote over the top, and finish with an extra sprinkle of lemon zest or hemp seeds if desired.

Pro Tip: These freeze and reheat well—make a double batch and store for busy mornings.

Avocado & Smoked Salmon Toast (GF)

Prep Time: 10 minutes

Servings: 2

2 slices gluten-free or grain-free bread (look for almond flour, cassava, or seed-based options without gums or refined starches)*

1 ripe avocado

Juice of ½ lemon

Pinch of sea salt

Pinch of red chili flakes (adjust to taste)

3–4 oz wild-caught smoked salmon

Handful of microgreens or arugula

Optional: 2 poached eggs

Optional: Extra virgin olive oil (for drizzling)

1. Toast your chosen GF bread until crisp but not dry. If using grain-free options, be gentle—they're often more delicate.

2. In a bowl, mash avocado with lemon juice, sea salt, and chili flakes. Spread generously over each slice of toast.

3. Layer smoked salmon over the avocado mash. Go for thin slices and fold them gently for texture.

4. Add a small handful of microgreens or arugula for crunch, color, and a bitter green anti-inflammatory punch.

5. Top with a freshly poached egg if you want extra protein and richness. Or drizzle with EVOO for added healthy fats and flavor.

Quick Tip:

This combo also works great on sweet potato slices or seed crackers if you're skipping bread entirely.

Coconut Yogurt Parfait

Prep Time: 5 minutes

Servings: 1 (easily doubled or batch-prepped)

¾ cup unsweetened coconut yogurt (look for live cultures and no added sugar)

½ kiwi, peeled and chopped

3–4 strawberries, chopped

1 tablespoon raw pumpkin seeds

1 teaspoon chia seeds

1 teaspoon cacao nibs

¼ teaspoon cinnamon

Dash of vanilla extract (optional)

1. In a small glass or bowl, spoon in half the coconut yogurt. Add a layer of chopped fruit and seeds.

2. Add remaining yogurt, then top with more fruit, pumpkin seeds, chia seeds, and cacao nibs.

3. Sprinkle cinnamon over the top and add a dash of vanilla for a dessert-like vibe without the sugar crash.

Pro Tips:

Want it sweeter? Add ½ tsp raw honey or a few chopped dates.

For a protein boost, mix in collagen powder or a spoonful of nut butter.

Chill it for 30 mins if you want the chia seeds to soften and thicken the mix slightly

Sautéed Veggie & Tofu Scramble

Prep Time: 10 minutes

Cook Time: 15 minutes

Servings: 2

1 block (about 14 oz) organic firm or extra-firm tofu (or tempeh)

1 small zucchini, chopped

½ cup mushrooms, sliced (shiitake, cremini, or button work great)

2 handfuls baby spinach

2 cloves garlic, minced

½ teaspoon turmeric

½ teaspoon ground cumin

½ teaspoon smoked paprika

Sea salt and black pepper, to taste

1 tablespoon avocado oil (or olive oil)

Optional toppings:

½ avocado, sliced

Drizzle of tahini or squeeze of lemon

1. Drain tofu and press it for 10–15 minutes to remove excess water. Then crumble it into bite-sized chunks using your hands or a fork. *(If using tempeh, chop into small cubes.)*

2. In a skillet, heat avocado oil over medium heat. Sauté zucchini and mushrooms for about 5–6 minutes, until softened and slightly browned. Add garlic and cook for 1 more minute.

3. Stir in the crumbled tofu and sprinkle with turmeric, cumin, smoked paprika, salt, and pepper. Mix well to evenly coat everything. Cook for another 5–7 minutes, stirring occasionally.

4. Toss in the spinach and let it wilt—about 1 minute.

5. Serve warm with sliced avocado or a drizzle of tahini. A squeeze of fresh lemon juice adds brightness.

Golden Milk Oats (Gluten-Free)

Prep Time: 5 minutes

Cook Time: 10 minutes

Servings: 2

1 cup gluten-free rolled oats

2 cups unsweetened almond milk or oat milk

½ teaspoon ground turmeric

½ teaspoon ground cinnamon

1–2 pinches freshly ground black pepper

2 fresh figs, sliced (or 3–4 dried, chopped)

2 tablespoons raw pistachios, roughly chopped

2 tablespoons almond butter

Optional: 1 teaspoon raw honey or date syrup (if extra sweetness is desired)

1. In a saucepan, combine oats and plant milk. Bring to a gentle simmer over medium heat, stirring occasionally.

2. Stir in turmeric, cinnamon, and black pepper. Continue to cook for about 8–10 minutes, until the oats are soft and creamy.

3. Divide the cooked oats between two bowls. Top with sliced figs, pistachios, and a generous dollop of almond butter.

4. Drizzle a touch of raw honey or date syrup over the top if you need a little extra sweetness.

Tips & Variations:

Use steel-cut oats for a chewier texture (increase cook time).

Add a splash of vanilla or grated fresh ginger for extra depth.

No figs? Use chopped apples, pears, or berries.

Batch-cook oats and reheat with a splash of extra milk throughout the week.

Leftovers for Breakfast (Yes, Really)

Prep Time: 5 minutes (or less)

Cook Time: 5 minutes (if adding an egg)

Servings: 1 (scale as needed)

1 cup leftover roasted veggies (broccoli, sweet potatoes, Brussels sprouts, carrots)

½ cup cooked wild rice, quinoa, or any grain-free base like cauliflower rice (optional)

1 small piece of leftover protein (wild-caught salmon, chicken, tempeh)

1 pasture-raised egg (sunny-side up or poached) or ½ avocado

2 tablespoons fermented veggies (e.g., kimchi, sauerkraut)

Drizzle of extra virgin olive oil or tahini (optional)

Sea salt, black pepper, chili flakes or lemon juice to taste

1. Warm your roasted veggies, rice, and protein in a skillet with a little olive oil—or eat them cold if you're in a rush.

2. Fry or poach an egg if you want a fresh, warm protein hit. Season with salt and pepper.

3. Arrange the reheated (or cold) veggies and protein in a bowl. Add the egg or sliced avocado on top.

4. Spoon kimchi or sauerkraut on the side. Drizzle with EVOO, tahini, or a squeeze of lemon if desired.

Tips:

Keep roasted veggie and grain mixes on hand throughout the week.

Change it up daily—different proteins, spices, or sauces.

Add leafy greens or sprouts for a fresh hit.

L U N CH

Bonus tip: Pair any of these with a cup of ginger tea or green tea to keep digestion smooth and inflammation even lower.

Wild Salmon Bowl with Turmeric Quinoa

Prep Time: 15 minutes

Cook Time: 20 minutes

Servings: 2

For the Bowl:

2 wild-caught salmon fillets (4–6 oz each)

1 cup quinoa, rinsed

2 cups water or low-sodium vegetable broth

1 teaspoon ground turmeric

1 tablespoon olive oil or avocado oil

1 cup broccoli florets (lightly steamed)

1 cup arugula

1 ripe avocado, sliced

1 tablespoon sesame seeds (optional)

For the Tahini-Lemon Dressing:

2 tablespoons tahini

Juice of 1 lemon

1 small garlic clove, minced

1–2 tablespoons warm water (to thin)

Pinch of sea salt and black pepper

1. In a saucepan, combine quinoa, water (or broth), and turmeric. Bring to a boil, then reduce to a simmer,

Cover, and cook for 15 minutes or until fluffy. Set aside.

2. Season fillets with sea salt and black pepper. Heat oil in a skillet over medium heat and cook salmon skin-side down for \~4–5 minutes, flip, and cook another 2–4 minutes, or until opaque and flakes easily. (Alternatively, bake at 375°F/190°C for 12–15 minutes.)*

3. Lightly steam for 3–4 minutes until just tender but still vibrant green.

4. Whisk together tahini, lemon juice, garlic, salt, pepper, and warm water until smooth and pourable.

5. Divide turmeric quinoa into two bowls. Top with steamed broccoli, arugula, salmon fillet, and avocado slices. Drizzle with tahini dressing and finish with a sprinkle of sesame seeds.

Lentil & Sweet Potato Curry

Prep Time: 10 minutes

Cook Time: 30 minutes

Servings: 4

1 tablespoon coconut oil or olive oil

1 small onion, finely chopped

2 cloves garlic, minced

1 tablespoon fresh ginger, grated

1 teaspoon ground turmeric

1 teaspoon ground cumin

1 cup red lentils, rinsed

1 medium sweet potato, peeled and cubed small

1 can (13.5 oz) full-fat coconut milk

2 cups vegetable broth or filtered water

2 cups chopped fresh spinach (or kale)

Sea salt and black pepper, to taste

Juice of ½ lime

To serve:

Steamed cauliflower rice or brown rice

Fresh cilantro

1. Heat oil in a large pot over medium heat. Add chopped onion and sauté for 3–4 minutes until translucent. Add garlic, ginger, turmeric, and cumin. Stir and cook for 1 more minute until fragrant.

2. Add red lentils, cubed sweet potatoes, coconut milk, and broth. Stir well. Bring to a gentle boil, then reduce heat to low and cover. Simmer for about 20–25 minutes, stirring occasionally, until lentils are soft and sweet potatoes are tender.

3. Stir in chopped spinach and cook for another 2–3 minutes until wilted. Season with sea salt, black pepper, and a squeeze of lime juice.

4. Spoon over cauliflower rice or brown rice. Garnish with fresh cilantro if desired.

Batch Tip:

This curry stores great in the fridge for 4 days or freezer for up to 2 months. Perfect for meal prep or doubling the recipe.

Mediterranean Chickpea Salad

Prep Time: 15 minutes

Servings: 2 as a main, 4 as a side

1½ cups cooked chickpeas (or 1 can, rinsed and drained)

1 cup cucumber, diced

1 cup cherry tomatoes, halved

¼ cup red onion, finely sliced or diced

¼ cup Kalamata olives, pitted and sliced

2 tablespoons fresh parsley, chopped

1 tablespoon fresh mint, chopped

Lemon-Olive Oil Dressing:

3 tablespoons extra virgin olive oil

Juice of 1 lemon

1 small garlic clove, finely grated or minced

Sea salt and black pepper to taste

Optional: ½ teaspoon dried oregano or sumac for extra Mediterranean punch

Optional Protein Add-Ons:

Grilled pasture-raised chicken breast (sliced)

Wild-caught grilled salmon (flaked)

1. In a small bowl or jar, whisk together olive oil, lemon juice, garlic, salt, pepper, and oregano/sumac if using.

2. In a large bowl, combine chickpeas, cucumber, tomatoes, red onion, and olives.

3. Pour the dressing over the salad and toss gently to combine. Add parsley and mint last for freshness.

4. Top with grilled chicken or salmon if using. Serve immediately or chill for 30 minutes to let the flavors meld

Make it work for you:

Store in the fridge for up to 3 days—great for batch prep.

Add greens like arugula or baby spinach to bulk it up.

Want it spicy? Add crushed red pepper flakes or a pinch of za'atar.

YOUR BODY DOES NOT HATE YOU, YOU'RE INFLAMED

Zucchini Noodles with Pesto & Grilled Chicken

Prep Time: 15 minutes

Cook Time: 15 minutes

Servings: 2

For the Zoodles + Toppings:

2–3 medium zucchinis, spiralized

1 cup cherry tomatoes, halved

1 handful arugula

2 organic chicken breasts

1 tablespoon extra-virgin olive oil

Sea salt and black pepper to taste

For the Homemade Pesto:

1 cup fresh basil leaves

1 garlic clove

¼ cup walnuts or pine nuts

¼ cup extra virgin olive oil

2 tablespoons nutritional yeast (for dairy-free) or grated pecorino/parmesan

Juice of ½ lemon

Sea salt to taste

Step 1: Make the Pesto

1. In a blender or food processor, combine basil, garlic, nuts, lemon juice, and nutritional yeast or cheese.

2. Pulse while slowly streaming in olive oil until smooth but still textured. Season with sea salt to taste. Set aside.

Step 2: Grill the Chicken

1. Season chicken breasts with salt and pepper.

2. Heat 1 tbsp olive oil in a grill pan or skillet over medium-high heat.

3. Grill chicken for 6–7 minutes per side, or until cooked through and juices run clear.

4. Let rest for 5 minutes, then slice thinly.

Step 3: Cook the Zoodles

1. In the same pan (wipe it down if needed), lightly sauté zucchini noodles for 1–2 minutes—just enough to warm and slightly soften them.

2. Add cherry tomatoes in the last 30 seconds to lightly blister them.

Step 4: Assemble

1. Toss the warm zoodles and tomatoes with 2–3 tablespoons of pesto (or more to taste).

2. Plate and top with sliced grilled chicken and a handful of fresh arugula.

Grilled Salmon Bowl with Greens & Tahini Dressing

Prep Time: 15 minutes

Cook Time: 10–12 minutes

Servings: 2

For the Salmon:

2 wild-caught salmon fillets (about 4–6 oz each)

1 tablespoon olive oil

1 teaspoon ground turmeric

2 cloves garlic, minced

Juice of ½ lemon

Sea salt and black pepper to taste

For the Bowl:

2 cups mixed greens (arugula, spinach, kale—lightly massaged if using kale)

1 cup cooked quinoa or 1½ cups cauliflower rice (lightly sautéed)

½ cup sliced cucumber

½ cup shredded carrots

1 avocado, sliced

Lemon-Tahini Dressing:

2 tablespoons tahini

Juice of 1 lemon

1 tablespoon olive oil

1 teaspoon maple syrup or raw honey

1–2 tablespoons water

Pinch of sea salt and black pepper

1. Prepare the Salmon:

In a small bowl, mix olive oil, turmeric, garlic, lemon juice, salt, and pepper.

Rub this marinade over the salmon fillets. Let it sit for 5–10 minutes while the grill or pan heats up.

Grill or pan-sear over medium heat for about 4–5 minutes per side, depending on thickness, until cooked through and flaky.

2. Whisk tahini, lemon juice, olive oil, and maple syrup (if using) in a small bowl. Add water gradually to reach desired consistency. Season with salt and pepper.

3. Build Your Bowl:

Divide greens between two bowls. Add quinoa or cauliflower rice as the base.

Top with cucumbers, carrots, avocado, and the cooked salmon.

Drizzle with lemon-tahini dressing just before serving.

Sardine & Avocado Salad Plate

Prep Time: 10 minutes

Servings: 1

1 can wild-caught sardines in olive oil (drained slightly, but keep some oil)

½ ripe avocado, sliced

2 cups arugula

½ cup cherry tomatoes, halved

2–3 radishes, thinly sliced

1 tablespoon raw pumpkin seeds

Lemon-Caper Vinaigrette:

1 tablespoon extra-virgin olive oil

1 tablespoon fresh lemon juice

½ teaspoon Dijon mustard

1 teaspoon capers, roughly chopped

Pinch of sea salt + freshly ground black pepper

1. Rinse and dry the arugula, slice the avocado, tomatoes, and radishes.

2. Whisk olive oil, lemon juice, mustard, capers, salt, and pepper in a small bowl until emulsified.

3. Arrange arugula as your base. Top with cherry tomatoes, radishes, and avocado slices. Add sardines on top or flaked into chunks.

4. Drizzle the vinaigrette over the salad, then sprinkle with pumpkin seeds for crunch and zinc.

5. Best eaten immediately. No cooking, no nonsense—just clean fuel.

Tip:

Upgrade it with a soft-boiled egg or a scoop of fermented veggies (like sauerkraut) for a probiotic bonus.

Thai-Inspired Rainbow Veggie Wraps

Prep Time: 20 minutes

Cook Time: 10 minutes (if grilling tofu or shrimp)

Servings: 2 (makes 4–6 wraps)

Wrap Base:

4–6 large collard green leaves (or rice paper wrappers)

Filling:

1 cup shredded carrots

1 cup thinly sliced bell peppers (any color)

1 cup shredded purple cabbage

1 avocado, sliced

1 cup grilled tofu or cooked shrimp

Cilantro, basil, or mint

Tahini-Lime Sauce:

2 tablespoons tahini or almond butter

1 tablespoon lime juice (freshly squeezed)

1 teaspoon tamari or coconut aminos

½ teaspoon grated fresh ginger

1–2 teaspoons warm water

1. Prep the wraps:

If using collard greens, blanch them in boiling water for 30 seconds to soften, then pat dry. Cut off the thickest part of the stem.

If using rice paper, soak one sheet at a time in warm water for 10–15 seconds until pliable.

2. Grill the protein:

For tofu: Slice into strips and grill or pan-sear with a touch of coconut or avocado oil for 3–5 minutes per side.

For shrimp: Cook in a pan over medium heat with sea salt and a splash of lime until pink and opaque (about 2–3 minutes per side).

3. Lay out your wrap base. Layer in a bit of each veggie, avocado, protein, and herbs. Be generous but don't overfill. Drizzle with tahini-lime sauce.

4. Fold the sides over, roll tightly like a burrito or spring roll, and slice in half if desired.

5. Serve with extra sauce on the side for dipping.

Cauliflower & Chickpea Curry Bowl

Prep Time: 10 minutes

Cook Time: 25 minutes

Servings: 4

1 tablespoon coconut oil or avocado oil

1 small yellow onion, finely chopped

3 cloves garlic, minced

1 tablespoon fresh ginger, grated

1 tablespoon curry powder

1 teaspoon ground turmeric

1 teaspoon ground cumin

1 head cauliflower, cut into small florets

1 can (15 oz) chickpeas, drained and rinsed

1 can (13.5 oz) full-fat coconut milk

1 cup crushed tomatoes (no added sugar or additives)

½ teaspoon sea salt or to taste

2 cups cooked quinoa or basmati rice

Fresh cilantro, chopped

Lime wedges

1. Heat oil in a large skillet or pot over medium heat. Add onion and sauté 3–4 minutes until soft. Stir in garlic and ginger; cook another 1 minute.

2. Add curry powder, turmeric, and cumin. Stir to coat the aromatics, releasing the oils and scent—about 30 seconds.

3. Add cauliflower florets, chickpeas, coconut milk, crushed tomatoes, and sea salt. Stir well and bring to a gentle simmer.

4. Cover and cook for 15–18 minutes, stirring occasionally, until cauliflower is soft but not mushy.

5. Spoon over cooked quinoa or rice. Garnish with chopped cilantro and a fresh squeeze of lime.

Seared Tuna & Avocado Nori Rolls

Prep Time: 15 minutes

Cook Time: 2–3 minutes

Servings: 2 (makes 4–6 rolls)

4–6 nori seaweed sheets

6 oz ahi tuna (sashimi-grade), seared or smoked salmon

½ avocado, thinly sliced

½ cucumber, julienned

½ cup shredded carrots

½ cup cauliflower rice (optional, lightly sautéed or raw)

Tamari or coconut aminos, for dipping

Optional: sesame seeds or a squeeze of lime for serving

1. If using ahi tuna, lightly season and sear in a hot pan for 30 seconds per side. Cool and slice into strips. (Skip this step if using smoked salmon.)

2. Julienne the cucumber and carrots, slice the avocado thinly, and lightly sauté the cauliflower rice if desired (no oil needed—just soften it slightly).

3. Place a sheet of nori rough-side-up on a clean surface. Near one edge, layer a few strips of tuna or salmon, a couple avocado slices, a small amount of cucumber, carrot, and cauliflower rice if using.

4. Roll the nori tightly like a sushi roll. Use a bit of water on the edge to seal the seam.

5. Use a very sharp knife to slice each roll into 4–6 bite-sized pieces. Wipe the blade clean between cuts for clean slices.

6. Serve with a small dish of tamari or coconut aminos, and garnish with sesame seeds or a squeeze of lime if you like.

Roasted Veggie & Hummus Plate

Prep Time: 10 minutes

Cook Time: 25–30 minutes

Servings: 2 (easily doubled for batch cooking)

For the roasted veggies:

1 zucchini, sliced into half-moons

1 small eggplant, cubed

2 carrots, cut into sticks

1 small head broccoli, broken into florets

2 tablespoons extra virgin olive oil

½ teaspoon sea salt

¼ teaspoon black pepper

Optional: pinch of smoked paprika or cumin

For the hummus (makes extra):

1 can chickpeas (or 1½ cups cooked), drained and rinsed

¼ cup tahini

2–3 garlic cloves, crushed

Juice of 1 lemon

2 tablespoons extra virgin olive oil

2–4 tablespoons water, to thin

Sea salt to taste

Optional: pinch of cumin or smoked paprika

Extras:

Sprouted seed crackers or sliced cucumber rounds

Fresh parsley, chopped

Extra lemon wedges

Extra virgin olive oil

1. Preheat oven to 400°F (200°C). Toss zucchini, eggplant, carrots, and broccoli in olive oil, salt, pepper, and spices (if using). Spread on a baking sheet and roast for 25–30 minutes, flipping halfway through, until golden and tender.

2. While veggies roast, blend all hummus ingredients in a food processor or high-speed blender. Adjust seasoning and add water to reach desired creaminess.

3. Divide roasted veggies between plates. Add a generous scoop of hummus to each. Serve with sprouted crackers or cucumber slices.

4. Drizzle with olive oil, sprinkle chopped parsley, and squeeze fresh lemon over everything.

Batch Cooking Tip:

Roast a double batch of veggies and keep them in the fridge for 3–4 days. Hummus also keeps well in an airtight container for up to a week.

M
A
I
N COURSE

YOUR BODY DOES NOT HATE YOU, YOU'RE INFLAMED

Herb-Crusted Wild Salmon with Garlic Greens

Prep Time: 10 minutes

Cook Time: 20 minutes

Servings: 2

For the Salmon:

2 wild-caught salmon fillets (4–6 oz each)

2 tablespoons extra virgin olive oil

2 tablespoons fresh parsley, finely chopped

1 tablespoon fresh dill, finely chopped

2 cloves garlic, minced

Zest of 1 lemon

Sea salt and black pepper to taste

Lemon wedges, for serving

For the Garlic Greens:

4 cups kale (or chard/spinach), chopped and destemmed

1 tablespoon olive oil

2 cloves garlic, thinly sliced

Splash of water or broth

Pinch of sea salt

Optional Side (Roasted Sweet Potatoes):

1 medium sweet potato, diced

1 tablespoon olive oil

Pinch of cinnamon and sea salt

1. Preheat oven to 400°F (200°C). Toss diced sweet potatoes in olive oil, cinnamon, and salt. Spread on a parchment-lined baking sheet and roast for 25–30 minutes, flipping halfway through. Start these first if including.

2. In a small bowl, mix olive oil, parsley, dill, garlic, and lemon zest. Pat the salmon dry, season with sea salt and pepper, and coat the top of each fillet with the herb mixture.

Place salmon skin-side down on a parchment-lined baking sheet. Bake at 400°F (200°C) for 12–15 minutes, depending on thickness, until it flakes easily with a fork.

3. While the salmon bakes, heat 1 tbsp olive oil in a skillet over medium heat. Add garlic slices and sauté until fragrant (about 1 minute). Add kale and a splash of water. Sauté 4–5 minutes until wilted but still vibrant. Season lightly with salt.

To Serve: Plate salmon with garlic greens on the side, add roasted sweet potatoes if desired, and squeeze a lemon wedge over the top. Serve warm.

Grass-Fed Lamb & Root Veggie Tagine

Prep Time: 15 minutes

Cook Time: 2 hours (stovetop or slow cooker)

Servings: 4

1.5 lbs grass-fed lamb shoulder or stew meat, cut into chunks

2 tablespoons extra virgin olive oil

1 large onion, diced

3 cloves garlic, minced

2 teaspoons ground turmeric

1 teaspoon ground cinnamon

1 teaspoon ground cumin

1 teaspoon ground ginger (or 1 tbsp fresh grated ginger)

Sea salt and black pepper, to taste

2 medium carrots, sliced

2 parsnips, chopped

1 large sweet potato, peeled and cubed

1 cup crushed tomatoes (no added sugar)

2 cups bone broth (beef or lamb)

Juice of ½ lemon

Handful of fresh mint, chopped

Optional garnish: fresh parsley or cilantro

For serving:

Cauliflower rice (light and low-carb) or cooked quinoa

1. Heat olive oil in a heavy-bottomed pot or Dutch oven over medium-high heat. Add lamb pieces in batches and brown on all sides. Set aside.

2. In the same pot, lower heat to medium. Add onion and cook until soft (about 5 minutes). Add garlic, turmeric, cinnamon, cumin, and ginger. Stir for 1 minute until fragrant.

3. Return lamb to the pot. Add carrots, parsnips, sweet potatoes, crushed tomatoes, and bone broth. Season with salt and pepper

4. Bring to a boil, then reduce to low. Cover and simmer for 1.5–2 hours, stirring occasionally, until lamb is tender and veggies are soft. Add lemon juice near the end.

Slow cooker option: Cook on low for 6–7 hours or high for 4 hours.

5. Taste and adjust seasoning. Stir in fresh mint before serving. Ladle over warm cauliflower rice or quinoa. Garnish with parsley or cilantro if desired.

YOUR BODY DOES NOT HATE YOU, YOU'RE INFLAMED

Coconut Turmeric Chicken Thighs

Prep Time: 10 minutes

Cook Time: 35–40 minutes

Servings: 4

6 bone-in, skin-on chicken thighs (pasture-raised if possible)

1 tablespoon coconut oil or avocado oil

1 small red onion, sliced

1 red bell pepper, sliced

3 cloves garlic, minced

1 tablespoon fresh grated turmeric (or 1 teaspoon ground turmeric)

1 teaspoon ground ginger

1 can (13.5 oz) full-fat coconut milk

Juice of 1 lime

2 cups fresh spinach (or chopped kale)

Sea salt and black pepper to taste

Optional: fresh cilantro or basil

For serving:

Cauliflower mash *(steamed cauliflower blended with olive oil and garlic) or Cooked wild rice

1. Heat oil in a large skillet or Dutch oven over medium-high heat. Season chicken thighs with salt and pepper. Sear skin-side down for 5–6 minutes until golden brown, flip and cook another 3–4 minutes. Remove and set aside.

2. In the same pan, lower heat to medium. Add onion, bell pepper, garlic, turmeric, and ginger. Sauté for 2–3 minutes until fragrant.

3. Pour in coconut milk and lime juice, scraping up any browned bits from the pan. Stir to combine.

4. Return chicken thighs to the pan, skin-side up. Cover and simmer on low for 25 minutes. Uncover for the last 5–10 minutes to thicken the sauce.

5. Stir in spinach (or kale) and simmer for another 2–3 minutes until wilted.

6. Plate over cauliflower mash or wild rice. Spoon sauce over the top. Garnish with fresh herbs if you like.

Veggie-Stuffed Acorn Squash with Tahini Drizzle

Prep Time: 15 minutes

Cook Time: 40 minutes

Servings: 2 (can double easily)

For the Squash:

1 medium acorn squash, halved and seeds removed

1 tablespoon olive oil

Sea salt and black pepper, to taste

For the Filling:

1 tablespoon olive oil

½ red onion, diced

2 cloves garlic, minced

1 cup mushrooms, chopped (shiitake or cremini are great)

2 cups kale, chopped and destemmed

¼ cup walnuts, roughly chopped

½ teaspoon thyme or rosemary (optional)

Sea salt and black pepper to taste

For the Tahini Drizzle:

2 tablespoons tahini

Juice of ½ lemon

1 tablespoon warm water (more as needed)

Pinch of sea salt

Optional: dash of garlic powder or cumin

1. Preheat oven to 400°F (200°C). Brush the cut sides of the squash with olive oil, sprinkle with salt and pepper, and place cut side down on a parchment-lined baking sheet. Roast for 35–40 minutes until flesh is tender and edges are caramelized.

2. Make the Filling:

While squash roasts, heat 1 tbsp olive oil in a skillet over medium heat.

Sauté onions for 3–4 minutes until translucent. Add garlic and cook 1 minute more.

Add mushrooms and cook until they release their moisture and start to brown (5–6 minutes).

Toss in chopped kale, cook until wilted (2–3 minutes). Stir in walnuts, thyme (if using), and season with salt and pepper. Remove from heat.

YOUR BODY DOES NOT HATE YOU, YOU'RE INFLAMED

3. In a small bowl, combine tahini, lemon juice, warm water, and seasonings. Stir until smooth. Add more water if needed to thin to a drizzle.

4. Assemble:

Flip roasted squash halves right side up. Fill each with the veggie-walnut mixture.

Drizzle generously with tahini sauce before serving.

Make it a meal: Serve with a side of quinoa or wild rice if you need more bulk.

Batch tip: Double the filling and freeze portions—it also works great stuffed in peppers or served over greens.

Baked Trout with Lemon-Herb Quinoa

Prep Time: 10 minutes

Cook Time: 20–25 minutes

Servings: 2

For the Trout:

2 trout fillets or 1 whole trout, cleaned and butterflied

1 tablespoon extra-virgin olive oil

1 lemon, thinly sliced

1 teaspoon fresh rosemary (or ½ tsp dried)

1 teaspoon fresh thyme (or ½ tsp dried)

Sea salt and black pepper to taste

For the Lemon-Herb Quinoa:

¾ cup uncooked quinoa (yields about 1.5 cups cooked)

1½ cups water or low-sodium vegetable broth

½ cucumber, finely diced

½ avocado, diced

¼ cup chopped fresh parsley

Juice of ½ lemon

1 tablespoon olive oil

Salt and pepper to taste

1. Cook the Quinoa:

Rinse quinoa thoroughly under cold water.

In a small saucepan, combine quinoa and water/broth. Bring to a boil, reduce to low, cover, and simmer for 15 minutes or until fluffy.

Remove from heat and let sit covered for 5 minutes. Fluff with a fork and allow to cool slightly.

2. Bake the Trout:

Preheat oven to 375°F (190°C).

Place trout fillets or whole fish on a baking sheet lined with parchment or foil.

Drizzle with olive oil, then season with salt, pepper, rosemary, and thyme.

Lay lemon slices over the top.

Bake for 15–20 minutes, depending on thickness, until the flesh flakes easily with a fork.

3. Finish the Quinoa:

In a bowl, combine cooked quinoa with cucumber, avocado, parsley, lemon juice, olive oil, and a pinch of salt and pepper.

Toss gently to mix without mashing the avocado.

4. Plate the trout alongside a generous scoop of quinoa salad. Serve warm or room temp.

Meal Prep Tip:

Double the quinoa portion—it keeps well for 3–4 days in the fridge and works great with chickpeas, grilled veggies, or other proteins.

Moroccan-Spiced Chickpea & Spinach Stew

Prep Time: 10 minutes

Cook Time: 25 minutes

Servings: 3–4

1 tablespoon extra virgin olive oil

1 small red onion, diced

2 medium carrots, chopped

3 cloves garlic, minced

1½ teaspoons ground cumin

1 teaspoon smoked paprika

½ teaspoon ground cinnamon

1 teaspoon ground turmeric

¼ teaspoon black pepper

Pinch of cayenne

1 (15 oz) can crushed tomatoes (no added sugar)

1½ cups cooked chickpeas (or 1 can, rinsed and drained)

2–3 cups fresh spinach (or 1 cup frozen spinach, thawed)

½ cup water or low-sodium veggie broth (as needed)

Sea salt to taste

Fresh lemon wedges

Optional Sides:

1 cup cooked millet or quinoa per serving

Fresh chopped parsley or cilantro for garnish

1. Heat olive oil in a large pot over medium heat. Add red onion and carrots. Cook for 5–6 minutes until softened.

2. Add garlic, cumin, paprika, cinnamon, turmeric, black pepper, and cayenne (if using). Stir constantly for 1–2 minutes until fragrant.

3. Pour in crushed tomatoes and chickpeas. Add a splash of water or broth to reach your desired stew consistency. Stir, bring to a simmer, cover partially, and cook for 15 minutes, stirring occasionally.

4. Stir in spinach and cook for 2–3 minutes until wilted. Adjust salt and spice to taste.

5. Ladle into bowls as-is or over a bed of quinoa or millet. Finish with a squeeze of fresh lemon and sprinkle of parsley or cilantro if you've got it.

Zucchini Lasagna (Grain & Dairy-Free)

Prep Time: 25 minutes

Cook Time: 40 minutes

Servings: 4–6

For the lasagna layers:

3 medium zucchinis, sliced lengthwise into thin strips (use a mandoline or sharp knife)

1 lb grass-fed ground beef or pasture-raised ground turkey

1 tablespoon olive oil

1 small onion, finely chopped

3 cloves garlic, minced

2 cups no-sugar-added crushed tomatoes or marinara sauce

1 teaspoon dried oregano

½ teaspoon sea salt

¼ teaspoon black pepper

For the cashew ricotta:

1 cup raw cashews (soaked 2–4 hrs or boiled for 10 mins)

2 tablespoons lemon juice

1 tablespoon olive oil

1 clove garlic

¼ cup water (plus more as needed)

1 tablespoon nutritional yeast

inch of sea salt

To finish:

Fresh basil leaves, torn

Olive oil drizzle

1. Slice zucchini into long, thin strips. Lightly salt and let them sit on paper towels for 10–15 mins to draw out moisture. Pat dry to prevent sogginess later.

2. Heat olive oil in a skillet over medium heat. Sauté onion until soft (about 5 mins), add garlic, then add ground beef or turkey. Cook through and season with salt, pepper, and oregano. Stir in the tomato sauce and let simmer for 10 minutes.

3. Drain cashews. Blend with lemon juice, garlic, olive oil, nutritional yeast, salt, and water until smooth and creamy. Add more water as needed for a spreadable texture.

4. Preheat oven to 375°F (190°C). In a baking dish, layer zucchini, meat sauce, and dollops of cashew ricotta. Repeat layers until all ingredients are used, finishing with sauce and ricotta on top.

5. Cover loosely with foil and bake for 30 minutes. Uncover and bake another 10 minutes until golden and bubbling.

6. Let it cool slightly. Top with fresh basil and a drizzle of olive oil before serving.

This one's freezer-friendly, meal-prep approved, and crowd-pleasing—even for folks who still eat the real thing.

Grilled Mackerel with Ginger Bok Choy

Prep Time: 10 minutes

Cook Time: 15 minutes

Servings: 2

For the mackerel:

2 whole mackerel (cleaned and gutted) or 2 fillets

2 cloves garlic, minced

Juice of ½ lemon

1 tablespoon olive oil

Sea salt and freshly cracked black pepper

Lemon wedges for serving

For the bok choy:

4 small heads of bok choy (or 2 large), halved or quartered

1 tablespoon sesame oil

1-inch fresh ginger, grated

1 tablespoon coconut aminos

1 teaspoon apple cider vinegar

Pinch of chili flakes

Optional sides:

1 cup steamed brown rice or cauliflower rice (choose based on your carb needs)

1. Pat the mackerel dry and brush with olive oil. Rub with garlic, lemon juice, salt, and pepper. Let it marinate while you prep the bok choy.

2. Heat a grill or grill pan over medium-high. Grill the fish for 4–5 minutes per side (fillets) or 6–7 minutes per side (whole fish), until skin is crispy and flesh flakes easily. Remove and rest for 2 minutes.

3. In a large skillet, heat sesame oil over medium heat. Add ginger and cook for 30 seconds until fragrant. Add bok choy, coconut aminos, and chili flakes. Stir-fry for 3–5 minutes until tender but still bright green. Finish with apple cider vinegar if using.

4. Serve grilled mackerel with the ginger bok choy and a side of rice or cauliflower rice. Garnish with fresh lemon wedges.

Batch tip: Grill multiple mackerel at once and use leftovers in salads or wraps the next day.

Slow Cooker Turmeric Chicken & Veggie Soup

Prep Time: 15 minutes

Cook Time: 6–8 hours on low (or 3–4 hours on high)

Servings: 4–6

.5 lbs boneless, skinless chicken thighs (pasture-raised if possible)

3 carrots, peeled and chopped

2 celery stalks, chopped

1 small onion, diced

3 cloves garlic, minced

1 teaspoon ground turmeric

½ teaspoon ground black pepper

1 teaspoon sea salt (or to taste)

4 cups bone broth (chicken or turkey, homemade or clean store-bought)

1–2 cups filtered water

2 cups chopped greens (chard, spinach, or kale)

Optional: juice of ½ lemon for brightness before serving

. Toss in chicken thighs, carrots, celery, onion, garlic, turmeric, pepper, salt, bone broth, and water.

2. Cook on low for 6–8 hours or high for 3–4 hours, until chicken is tender and veggies are soft.

3. Remove chicken with tongs, shred with two forks, and return it to the pot. Stir well.

4. About 5–10 minutes before serving, stir in chopped greens until wilted. (Spinach goes in last-minute; chard or kale can simmer a bit longer.)

5. Taste and adjust seasoning. Add lemon juice if desired. Serve hot.

Meal Prep Tip:

Let it cool and store in glass containers in the fridge (up to 4 days) or freezer (up to 3 months). Reheat gently on the stove—never microwave bone broth if you want to preserve its integrity.

Eggplant & Lentil Curry

Prep Time: 10 minutes

Cook Time: 30–35 minutes

Servings: 4

1 medium eggplant, cut into ½-inch cubes

¾ cup red lentils, rinsed well

1 tablespoon coconut oil or olive oil

1 small onion, diced

3 cloves garlic, minced

1 tablespoon fresh grated ginger (or 1 tsp ground ginger)

1 tablespoon curry powder (choose a blend without additives)

1 teaspoon ground turmeric

½ teaspoon ground cumin

½ teaspoon sea salt

1 (14 oz) can crushed tomatoes (no added sugar)

1 (14 oz) can full-fat coconut milk

1½ cups water or veggie broth

Fresh cilantro, chopped

2 tablespoons raw pumpkin seeds (pepitas), toasted if desired

1. Heat oil in a large pot over medium heat. Add onion, garlic, and ginger. Sauté for 2–3 minutes until fragrant and translucent.

2. Stir in curry powder, turmeric, and cumin. Toast for 1 minute to bloom the spices.

3. Toss in the cubed eggplant, crushed tomatoes, coconut milk, and water/broth. Stir to combine.

4. Stir in rinsed red lentils. Bring everything to a gentle boil, then reduce heat and simmer uncovered for 25–30 minutes, stirring occasionally.

5. Lentils should be tender and eggplant soft. Add a splash of water if it thickens too much.

6. Add sea salt and adjust spices as needed.

7. Spoon into bowls. Top with fresh chopped cilantro and pumpkin seeds for crunch.

Make it a meal:

Pair with steamed cauliflower rice or a scoop of quinoa. Stores great in the fridge for 3–4 days and freezes well

Bison & Veggie Skillet

Prep Time: 10 minutes

Cook Time: 15 minutes

Servings: 2

1 tablespoon extra-virgin olive oil or avocado oil

½ pound ground grass-fed bison

2 cloves garlic, minced

½ red onion, diced

1 zucchini, chopped

1 cup mushrooms, sliced

2 cups kale, chopped (destemmed)

½ teaspoon smoked paprika

½ teaspoon ground cumin

1 tablespoon coconut aminos

Sea salt and freshly ground black pepper, to taste

Optional toppings:

½ avocado, sliced

1–2 fried pasture-raised eggs

1. Heat oil in a large skillet over medium heat. Add garlic and onions, sauté 2–3 minutes until soft.

2. Add ground bison. Cook for 5–7 minutes, breaking it up with a spatula, until browned and mostly cooked through.

3. Toss in zucchini and mushrooms. Stir well and cook for another 5–6 minutes until softened.

4. Stir in kale, smoked paprika, cumin, coconut aminos, and salt/pepper. Cook 1–2 minutes more, just until the kale wilts and everything is coated in flavor.

5. Plate and top with sliced avocado or a fried egg if desired.

Coconut Curry Shrimp & Veggies

Prep Time: 10 minutes

Cook Time: 20 minutes

Servings: 2

. 1 lb wild-caught shrimp, peeled and deveined

1 tablespoon coconut oil

2 cloves garlic, minced

1 tablespoon fresh ginger, grated

1 tablespoon curry powder (look for a blend with turmeric)

1 can (13.5 oz) full-fat coconut milk

Juice of ½ lime (plus wedges for serving)

1 red bell pepper, sliced thin

1 cup broccoli florets

2 cups spinach or baby kale

Sea salt and black pepper to taste

Optional: crushed red pepper flakes for heat

Serve with: ½ cup cooked jasmine rice or 1 cup cauliflower rice per serving

1. Heat coconut oil in a large skillet over medium heat. Add garlic and ginger, sauté for 1 minute until fragrant.

2. Stir in curry powder and cook for another 30 seconds. Pour in coconut milk and lime juice. Bring to a simmer.

3. Toss in bell pepper and broccoli. Simmer for 5–7 minutes until just tender.

4. Add shrimp to the skillet. Simmer 3–5 minutes, stirring occasionally, until shrimp turn pink and are cooked through.

5. Stir in spinach or baby kale, let it wilt into the curry (1–2 minutes). Season with sea salt and black pepper to taste.

6. Spoon curry over jasmine or cauliflower rice. Garnish with lime wedges and red pepper flakes if desired.

Stuffed Bell Peppers (Quinoa + Turkey)

Prep Time: 15 minutes

Cook Time: 30–35 minutes

Servings: 4 (1 pepper per serving)

4 large bell peppers (any color), tops sliced off and seeds removed

1 lb ground turkey (pasture-raised if possible)

1 cup cooked quinoa

2 cups chopped spinach (fresh or frozen, squeezed dry)

2 cloves garlic, minced

1 small red onion, finely diced

1 tablespoon olive oil

1 teaspoon dried oregano or Italian herb blend

½ teaspoon turmeric

¼ teaspoon black pepper

Sea salt to taste

Optional toppings:

Avocado cream (blended avocado + lime + garlic)

Dairy-free pesto (basil, olive oil, garlic, lemon, nuts/seeds)

1. To 375°F (190°C). Lightly grease a baking dish.

2. Cook quinoa if you haven't already (1 part quinoa to 2 parts water, simmered for \~15 minutes).

3. In a skillet, heat olive oil. Add onion and garlic, cook for 2–3 minutes until softened. Add ground turkey, turmeric, herbs, pepper, and salt. Cook until browned and fully cooked through. Stir in spinach and cooked quinoa, mix until everything is heated through and well-combined.

4. Place hollowed peppers upright in a baking dish. Spoon the turkey-quinoa mixture into each one, packing tightly.

5. Cover with foil and bake for 25 minutes. Uncover and bake for another 5–10 minutes until the peppers are soft and the tops are golden.

6. Drizzle with avocado cream or a spoonful of dairy-free pesto before serving.

Grilled Chicken with Chimichurri & Roasted Veggies

Prep Time: 15 minutes

Cook Time: 30–35 minutes

Servings: 2

For the Chicken:

4 organic, boneless skinless chicken thighs

1 tablespoon olive oil

½ teaspoon sea salt

½ teaspoon black pepper

½ teaspoon smoked paprika

For the Chimichurri:

1 cup fresh parsley, finely chopped

2–3 garlic cloves, minced

¼ cup extra virgin olive oil

2 tablespoons red wine vinegar or apple cider vinegar

½ teaspoon sea salt

Pinch of crushed red pepper flakes

For the Roasted Veggies:

1 cup Brussels sprouts, halved

1 medium sweet potato, diced

½ red onion, sliced

1–2 tablespoons olive oil

Sea salt and pepper, to taste

½ teaspoon turmeric

1. Preheat oven to 400°F (200°C). Toss Brussels sprouts, sweet potatoes, and red onion with olive oil, salt, pepper, and turmeric. Spread on a baking sheet in a single layer and roast for 30–35 minutes, flipping halfway through.

2. While veggies roast, mix parsley, garlic, olive oil, vinegar, salt, and red pepper flakes in a small bowl. Let it sit at room temp so the flavors meld.

3. Heat a grill pan or outdoor grill to medium-high. Rub chicken thighs with olive oil, salt, pepper, and paprika. Grill 4–5 minutes per side or until fully cooked (internal temp 165°F/74°C). Let rest for 5 minutes.

4. Plate the roasted veggies. Top the grilled chicken with a generous spoonful of chimichurri.

Cauliflower Tabbouleh with Wild Salmon

Prep Time: 15 minutes

Cook Time: 12–15 minutes

Servings: 2

For the Tabbouleh:

2 cups cauliflower rice (store-bought or pulsed from 1 medium head)

1 cup finely chopped parsley

¼ cup chopped fresh mint

1 cup diced cucumber

¾ cup diced tomato (roma or cherry)

2 tablespoons extra virgin olive oil

Juice of 1 lemon

Sea salt and black pepper to taste

For the Salmon:

2 wild-caught salmon fillets (4–6 oz each)

1 tablespoon olive oil or avocado oil

Sea salt and black pepper

Optional: pinch of paprika or garlic powder

Tahini Drizzle (optional but awesome):

2 tablespoons tahini

1 tablespoon lemon juice

1 tablespoon water

Pinch of sea salt and cumin

1. Make the tabbouleh:

If using a whole cauliflower, pulse florets in a food processor until rice-like.

In a large bowl, toss cauliflower rice with parsley, mint, cucumber, tomato, olive oil, lemon juice, salt, and pepper. Let it chill while you cook the salmon.

2. Cook the salmon:

Heat oil in a skillet over medium heat.

Season salmon with salt, pepper, and optional spices.

Cook skin-side down first for about 4–5 minutes. Flip and cook another 3–4 minutes, or until cooked through and flakey.

Alternatively, bake at 400°F (200°C) for 12–14 minutes.

3. Whisk all drizzle ingredients in a small bowl until smooth. Add more water for a thinner texture.

4. Divide the tabbouleh between two plates. Top each with a salmon fillet and a light drizzle of tahini if using.

Thai-Inspired Chicken Lettuce Wraps

Prep Time: 10 minutes

Cook Time: 15 minutes

Servings: 2–3

1 lb ground chicken (organic or pasture-raised preferred)

1 tablespoon avocado oil or coconut oil

2 cloves garlic, minced

1 tablespoon fresh ginger, minced or grated

3 scallions, thinly sliced (separate whites and greens)

2 tablespoons coconut aminos (soy-free, low sodium)

Juice of 1 lime

Sea salt and black pepper to taste

1–2 heads of butter lettuce, iceberg, or romaine (for cups)

Toppings:

½ cup shredded carrots

¼ cup raw or dry-roasted cashews, chopped

Optional: chopped cilantro, extra lime wedges, crushed red pepper

1. Heat oil in a skillet over medium heat. Add garlic, ginger, and the white parts of scallions. Sauté for 1–2 minutes until fragrant.

2. Add ground chicken. Break it up with a spatula and cook until fully browned and no longer pink (about 7–10 minutes).

3. Stir in coconut aminos, lime juice, sea salt, and pepper. Let it simmer for 2 more minutes so the flavors absorb.

4. While the chicken cooks, gently separate and rinse the lettuce leaves. Pat dry and set aside.

5. Spoon the chicken mixture into lettuce cups. Top with shredded carrots, chopped cashews, green scallions, and optional extras.

Pro Tip:

Batch the chicken ahead of time and store it in the fridge. You can reheat and build wraps on the fly for quick lunches or dinners.

Hearty Veggie & White Bean Soup

Prep Time: 15 minutes

Cook Time: 30 minutes

Servings: 4

1 tablespoon extra-virgin olive oil

1 small yellow onion, diced

2 carrots, diced

2 celery stalks, diced

3 cloves garlic, minced

1 medium zucchini, chopped

1½ cups cooked cannellini beans (or 1 can, drained and rinsed)

4 cups bone broth or high-quality vegetable stock

2 cups chopped kale (remove tough stems)

1 teaspoon dried thyme

1 teaspoon dried rosemary

Sea salt and black pepper to taste

Optional: juice of ½ lemon for brightness

To Serve:

Gluten-free toast or seed crackers

Fresh chopped parsley or drizzle of olive oil on top (optional)

1. Heat olive oil in a large soup pot over medium heat. Add onion, carrots, and celery. Cook for 5–7 minutes until softened.

2. Stir in garlic and zucchini. Cook for another 2–3 minutes until fragrant.

3. Add cannellini beans, thyme, rosemary, and broth. Bring to a boil, then reduce to a simmer. Cook uncovered for 15–20 minutes, stirring occasionally.

4. Stir in kale during the last 5 minutes of cooking. Let it wilt but stay vibrant.

5. Taste and adjust seasoning with sea salt and pepper. Add lemon juice if using.

6. Ladle into bowls and serve with gluten-free toast or seed crackers. Add fresh herbs or a drizzle of olive oil if desired.

Turkey Meatballs in Spicy Tomato Sauce

Prep Time: 15 minutes

Cook Time: 30 minutes

Servings: 4

For the meatballs:

1 lb ground turkey (pasture-raised if possible)

2 garlic cloves, minced

2 tablespoons ground flaxseed

2 tablespoons fresh parsley, chopped (or 1 tsp dried)

1 teaspoon dried oregano

½ teaspoon sea salt

¼ teaspoon black pepper

Optional: 1 egg (or 1 tbsp more flaxseed + 3 tbsp water for binder)

Olive oil for baking or pan-searing

For the sauce:

1 tablespoon extra virgin olive oil

2–3 cloves garlic, minced

1 (28 oz) can crushed tomatoes (no added sugar)

1 teaspoon dried basil

1 teaspoon dried oregano

½ teaspoon red chili flakes

Sea salt and pepper to taste

Optional: splash of balsamic vinegar or pinch of coconut sugar to balance acidity

Serving options:

Zucchini noodles (zoodles)

Roasted spaghetti squash

Cooked quinoa

1. Preheat oven to 400°F (200°C). In a bowl, mix ground turkey, garlic, flaxseed, herbs, salt, and pepper. Add the egg (or flax egg alternative) if using. Form into 1.5-inch balls.

2. Place meatballs on a parchment-lined baking sheet and bake for 18–20 minutes until cooked through.

   OR heat a drizzle of olive oil in a skillet and sear the meatballs on all sides, then finish cooking them in the sauce.

3. While the meatballs cook, heat olive oil in a large pan over medium. Sauté garlic for 30 seconds, then add crushed tomatoes, basil, oregano, chili flakes, and seasoning. Let simmer for 10–15 minutes.

4. Add cooked meatballs to the sauce. Simmer for another 5–10 minutes so the flavors marry.

5. Spoon the meatballs and sauce over a bed of zucchini noodles, spaghetti squash, or quinoa.

Miso-Glazed Cod with Broccoli & Shiitake Stir-Fry

Prep Time: 15 minutes

Cook Time: 20 minutes

Servings: 2

For the cod:

2 wild-caught cod fillets (4–6 oz each)

2 tablespoons white or yellow miso paste

1 tablespoon grated fresh ginger

1 teaspoon toasted sesame oil

1 tablespoon rice vinegar or lime juice

1 teaspoon raw honey or date syrup

For the stir-fry:

1 tablespoon toasted sesame oil

1 cup shiitake mushrooms, sliced

1½ cups broccoli florets

1 cup bok choy, chopped

1–2 tablespoons coconut aminos (soy sauce alternative)

1 clove garlic, minced

Pinch of sea salt and black pepper

Optional side:

½ cup cooked millet or black (forbidden) rice per person

1. In a small bowl, whisk together miso, ginger, sesame oil, rice vinegar (or lime), and honey/date syrup. Brush over cod fillets and let marinate in the fridge for 10–15 minutes while you prep the veggies.

2. Preheat oven to 375°F (190°C). Place cod on a parchment-lined baking sheet and bake for 12–15 minutes, or until the fish flakes easily with a fork.

3. While cod bakes, heat sesame oil in a large skillet or wok over medium heat. Add mushrooms and broccoli; stir-fry for 3–4 minutes. Add bok choy, garlic, and coconut aminos. Cook another 3–5 minutes until veggies are just tender but still vibrant.

4. Serve the baked cod on a bed of stir-fried veggies. Optional: spoon over a scoop of warm millet or black rice.

Pro Tip:

Make extra miso glaze—it also works brilliantly on salmon, tofu, or roasted veggies. Want to turn this into a meal prep version? Just ask.

SOUPS AND STEWS

Pro tip: Make double batches and freeze in glass containers or silicone trays for easy pull-and-heat meals.

Golden Turmeric Chicken Soup

Prep Time: 15 minutes

Cook Time: 30 minutes

Servings: 4

1 tablespoon extra-virgin olive oil or coconut oil

1 small onion, diced

2 carrots, peeled and sliced

2 celery stalks, sliced

3 cloves garlic, minced

1 tablespoon fresh grated ginger or 1 tsp ground

1 tablespoon fresh grated turmeric or 1 tsp ground

¼ teaspoon black pepper

½ teaspoon sea salt or to taste

4 cups bone broth (chicken or turkey)

1 cup cooked, shredded organic chicken (leftover or pre-poached)

¼ cup full-fat coconut milk

Optional: 2 cups spinach or chopped kale

Optional garnish: fresh parsley or cilantro

1. In a large soup pot, heat oil over medium heat. Add onions, carrots, and celery. Cook for 5–7 minutes until softened.

2. Stir in garlic, ginger, turmeric, black pepper, and salt. Cook for 1–2 minutes until fragrant.

3. Pour in the bone broth. Bring to a gentle boil, then reduce to a simmer. Cook uncovered for 15–20 minutes until vegetables are tender.

4. Stir in the shredded chicken and coconut milk. Let it warm through for about 5 minutes.

5. Add spinach or kale during the last 2–3 minutes of cooking, just until wilted.

6. Adjust seasoning if needed. Ladle into bowls and top with fresh herbs if you like.

Spiced Lentil & Spinach Stew

Prep Time: 10 minutes

Cook Time: 25 minutes

Servings: 4

1 tablespoon extra-virgin olive oil or coconut oil

1 small red onion, diced

3 cloves garlic, minced

1 teaspoon ground cumin

1 teaspoon ground coriander

1 teaspoon ground turmeric

1 cup red lentils, rinsed

1 can (14 oz) fire-roasted diced tomatoes

1 can (13.5 oz) full-fat coconut milk

2 cups low-sodium vegetable broth or water

3 cups fresh spinach, chopped

½ teaspoon sea salt (or to taste)

Fresh ground black pepper

For topping:

Fresh chopped cilantro

Lime wedges

1. In a large pot, heat the oil over medium heat. Add onion and cook 3–4 minutes until soft. Add garlic, cumin, coriander, and turmeric. Stir for 1 minute until fragrant.

2. Stir in rinsed red lentils, fire-roasted tomatoes, coconut milk, and broth. Bring to a gentle boil, then reduce heat to simmer.

3. Cover and cook for 15–20 minutes, stirring occasionally, until lentils are soft and the stew thickens.

4. Stir in chopped spinach and cook another 2–3 minutes until wilted. Season with salt and pepper to taste.

5. Ladle into bowls, top with fresh cilantro and a good squeeze of lime.

Butternut Squash & Ginger Soup

Prep Time: 15 minutes

Cook Time: 35 minutes

Servings: 4

1 medium butternut squash (about 2½ to 3 lbs), peeled, seeded, and cubed

1 tablespoon extra-virgin olive oil

1 medium yellow onion, chopped

3 cloves garlic, minced

1 tablespoon fresh ginger, grated or finely chopped

3 cups bone broth or vegetable broth (low-sodium, clean ingredients)

½ cup coconut cream or full-fat coconut milk

½ teaspoon ground cinnamon

¼ teaspoon ground nutmeg

Sea salt and black pepper to taste

Optional toppings: pumpkin seeds, chopped herbs, swirl of coconut cream

1. Preheat oven to 400°F (200°C). Spread cubed squash on a baking sheet, drizzle with olive oil, and roast for 25–30 minutes or until soft and golden on the edges.

2. In a large pot, heat a splash of olive oil over medium heat. Add onions and sauté for 5–6 minutes until translucent. Add garlic and ginger, cook for another 1–2 minutes until fragrant.

3. Add roasted squash to the pot with sautéed aromatics. Pour in broth and bring to a simmer for 5 minutes. Use an immersion blender to blend until smooth, or transfer carefully to a high-speed blender in batches.

4. Return to pot (if blended externally). Stir in coconut cream, cinnamon, nutmeg, salt, and pepper. Simmer gently for 5 more minutes to let flavors meld.

5. Ladle into bowls and garnish with your favorite toppings (toasted pumpkin seeds, parsley, swirl of coconut cream, etc.).

Wild Salmon & Seaweed Miso Soup

Prep Time: 10 minutes

Cook Time: 15 minutes

Servings: 2 large bowls

4 cups filtered water or low-sodium vegetable broth

2 tablespoons organic, unpasteurized miso paste (white or yellow)

1 tablespoon dried wakame seaweed

½ cup sliced shiitake mushrooms (fresh or dried & rehydrated)

1 cup baby bok choy, chopped

½ block organic tofu, cubed (firm or silken, your choice)

1 wild-caught salmon fillet (about 4–5 oz), skin removed, cut into bite-sized chunks

2 green onions, sliced thin

Optional: 1 teaspoon tamari or coconut aminos

Optional garnish: sesame seeds, chili flakes, or microgreens

1. In a bowl, soak wakame in warm water for 5 minutes until expanded. Drain and set aside.

2. Bring the water or broth to a simmer (not a full boil) in a medium pot. Add shiitake mushrooms and cook for 5–7 minutes until softened.

3. Add the salmon chunks and simmer gently for about 4 minutes until just cooked through. Don't boil—it keeps the texture tender and nutrients intact.

4. Toss in bok choy and tofu cubes. Cook another 2–3 minutes until greens are wilted.

5. Turn off the heat. In a small bowl, whisk miso paste with a bit of hot broth to dissolve. Stir this into the pot **after** removing from heat to preserve probiotics.

6. Add wakame and green onions. Optional splash of tamari or coconut aminos for added depth. Ladle into bowls and top with garnishes if using.

Pro Tip:

This soup keeps in the fridge for 2–3 days but add the miso and green onions fresh each time to retain their benefits.

Hearty Sweet Potato & Kale Stew

Prep Time: 15 minutes

Cook Time: 30–35 minutes

Servings: 4

1 tablespoon extra-virgin olive oil

1 medium yellow onion, diced

2 cloves garlic, minced

2 medium carrots, sliced

2 medium sweet potatoes, peeled and cubed

1 teaspoon smoked paprika

1 teaspoon dried rosemary (or 1 tbsp fresh)

Sea salt and black pepper to taste

4 cups low-sodium vegetable broth

1½ cups cooked chickpeas or lentils (or 1 can, rinsed)

3 cups chopped kale (destemmed)

Optional: pinch of crushed red pepper for heat, squeeze of lemon before serving

1. In a large pot, heat olive oil over medium heat. Add onion and carrots and sauté for 5 minutes until softened. Stir in garlic and cook for another 1–2 minutes until fragrant.

2. Stir in sweet potatoes, smoked paprika, rosemary, sea salt, and black pepper. Cook for 1–2 minutes to let the spices bloom.

3. Pour in the broth and bring to a boil. Reduce heat to low and simmer uncovered for 20 minutes, or until sweet potatoes are tender.

4. Stir in the chickpeas or lentils and chopped kale. Simmer another 5–10 minutes until kale is wilted and everything is well combined.

5. Adjust seasoning as needed. Add crushed red pepper for kick or a squeeze of lemon juice for brightness before serving.

Thai Coconut Curry Soup

Prep Time: 15 minutes

Cook Time: 20 minutes

Servings: 4

1 tablespoon coconut oil or avocado oil

1 small onion, thinly sliced

3 garlic cloves, minced

1 tablespoon fresh ginger, grated

2 teaspoons red curry paste (look for a clean version—no added sugar or MSG)

1 stalk lemongrass, smashed and chopped (or 1 tsp lemongrass paste)

1 can (13.5 oz) full-fat coconut milk

3 cups low-sodium vegetable or bone broth

1 tablespoon coconut aminos or gluten-free tamari

½ pound wild shrimp, peeled and deveined

1 cup mushrooms, sliced (shiitake or cremini work great)

1 cup bok choy, chopped

1 carrot, julienned or thinly sliced

Juice of 1 fresh lime

Handful of fresh cilantro leaves

Optional toppings:

Sliced chili or red pepper flakes for heat

Extra lime wedges

Mung bean sprouts or microgreens

1. In a large pot over medium heat, warm the coconut oil. Add onion, garlic, and ginger. Sauté for 3–4 minutes until softened.

2. Stir in red curry paste and lemongrass. Cook for 1–2 minutes to release the aroma.

3. Pour in coconut milk and broth. Stir in coconut aminos or tamari if using. Bring to a gentle simmer.

4. Add mushrooms, carrots, and bok choy. Simmer for 5 minutes. Then add shrimp and simmer another 3–5 minutes until shrimp are opaque and cooked through.

5. Remove from heat. Stir in fresh lime juice and sprinkle in cilantro.

6. Ladle into bowls and garnish with optional toppings. Best enjoyed fresh and hot.

Gut-Healing Bone Broth & Veggie Soup

Prep Time: 15 minutes

Cook Time: 30 minutes

Servings: 4

6 cups homemade bone broth (chicken, beef, or turkey)

2 carrots, sliced

2 celery stalks, diced

1 zucchini, chopped

1 leek, white and light green parts sliced thin

2 cups fresh spinach

2 cloves garlic, minced

1 teaspoon turmeric powder (or 1-inch fresh turmeric, grated)

1 teaspoon dried thyme

1 tablespoon olive oil or ghee

Sea salt and black pepper to taste

Optional: 1–2 cups shredded cooked chicken or turkey

1. In a large soup pot, heat olive oil or ghee over medium heat. Add garlic, turmeric, and leeks. Sauté 2–3 minutes until soft and fragrant.

2. Toss in carrots, celery, zucchini, and thyme. Cook another 5 minutes, stirring occasionally.

3. Add the broth and bring to a light boil. Reduce heat and let it simmer gently for about 20 minutes, or until veggies are tender.

4. Add spinach and shredded chicken or turkey if using. Simmer another 5 minutes until greens are wilted and meat is heated through.

5. Add sea salt and freshly ground black pepper to taste. Serve warm, and feel your insides thank you.

Moroccan Chickpea & Tomato Stew

Prep Time: 10 minutes

Cook Time: 25–30 minutes

Servings: 4

1 tablespoon extra-virgin olive oil

1 medium onion, diced

3 garlic cloves, minced

1 red bell pepper, diced

1 medium zucchini, chopped

2 carrots, diced

1½ cups cooked chickpeas (or 1 can, drained and rinsed)

1 can (14.5 oz) fire-roasted diced tomatoes

1 cup vegetable broth or filtered water

1 teaspoon ground cumin

1 teaspoon ground turmeric

½ teaspoon ground cinnamon

½ teaspoon smoked paprika

Sea salt and black pepper to taste

Juice of ½ lemon

Fresh parsley, chopped

Lemon wedges

1. In a large pot, heat olive oil over medium heat. Add onions and garlic. Cook for 2–3 minutes until fragrant and translucent.

2. Stir in bell pepper, zucchini, and carrots. Sauté for 5 minutes until veggies start to soften.

3. Add cumin, turmeric, and cinnamon, smoked paprika, salt, and black pepper. Stir well to coat the vegetables in the spices.

4. Add chickpeas, fire-roasted tomatoes, and broth. Stir, bring to a boil, then reduce heat and simmer uncovered for 15–20 minutes until vegetables are tender and stew thickens.

5. Squeeze in lemon juice, taste, and adjust seasoning if needed.

6. Ladle into bowls, garnish with chopped parsley, and serve with extra lemon wedges on the side.

Mushroom & Wild Rice Soup

Prep Time: 15 minutes

Cook Time: 45 minutes

Servings: 4

1 tablespoon extra-virgin olive oil or avocado oil

1 medium yellow onion, diced

2 celery stalks, chopped

3 cloves garlic, minced

3 cups mixed mushrooms (shiitake, cremini, oyster), sliced

¾ cup uncooked wild rice, rinsed

4 cups vegetable broth (low-sodium, clean label)

1 cup full-fat coconut milk

1 teaspoon fresh thyme leaves (or ½ tsp dried)

½ teaspoon black pepper

Sea salt to taste

Optional: squeeze of lemon at the end for brightness

1. Heat oil in a large pot over medium heat. Add onion and celery, and cook 5–6 minutes until soft and fragrant.

2. Stir in the garlic and mushrooms. Sauté 7–10 minutes, letting mushrooms release moisture and develop flavor.

3. Pour in the wild rice and vegetable broth. Bring to a boil, then reduce to a simmer. Cover and cook 35–40 minutes, until rice is tender.

4. Stir in coconut milk, thyme, black pepper, and salt to taste. Simmer uncovered another 5 minutes to let flavors meld.

5. Optional: Add a squeeze of lemon before serving to brighten it up. Ladle into bowls and enjoy warm.

Pro Tip:

This soup stores beautifully. Make a double batch and freeze half for those "no energy but want to eat clean" days.

YOUR BODY DOES NOT HATE YOU, YOU'RE INFLAMED

SIBO-Friendly Zucchini Basil Soup

Prep Time: 10 minutes

Cook Time: 15 minutes

Servings: 2–3

2 tablespoons garlic-infused olive oil (use oil only, no garlic pieces – low-FODMAP friendly)

4 medium zucchinis, chopped

1 tablespoon fresh ginger, grated (or ½ tsp ground ginger)

1½ cups bone broth (or use vegetable broth for plant-based option)

½ cup full-fat coconut milk (BPA-free canned is best)

½ cup fresh basil leaves, packed

Optional: 1 scoop collagen powder

Sea salt and freshly ground black pepper, to taste

Optional toppings: drizzle of garlic oil, chopped chives, or microgreens

1. In a medium pot, heat the garlic-infused olive oil over medium heat. Add chopped zucchini and ginger. Sauté for 5–6 minutes until zucchini begins to soften.

2. Pour in bone broth and bring to a simmer. Cook uncovered for 8–10 minutes until zucchini is tender.

3. Remove from heat. Add basil and coconut milk. Blend using an immersion blender right in the pot, or transfer carefully to a blender. Blend until silky smooth.

4. Stir in collagen powder if using. Season with sea salt and black pepper to taste.

5. Pour into bowls and top with a swirl of garlic oil, fresh herbs, or a few pumpkin seeds for crunch.

Pro tip: Make double batches and freeze in glass containers or silicone trays for easy pull-and-heat meals.

S
A
L
A
D
S & DRESSINGS

- Avoid store-bought unless it's made with olive oil or avocado oil and no weird additives.
- Batch it. Make 1–2 dressings a week in glass jars for quick drizzle-and-go meals.
- Add fresh herbs or spices to level up the anti-inflammatory power: turmeric, oregano, parsley, garlic, basil, etc.

Wild Salmon Power Salad

Prep Time: 10 minutes

Cook Time: 10–15 minutes (if cooking salmon fresh)

Servings: 2

For the Salad:

4–5 cups mixed leafy greens (arugula, spinach, romaine, etc.)

1 wild-caught salmon fillet (about 6–8 oz)

½ avocado, sliced

½ cucumber, thinly sliced

½ cup shredded carrot

2 tablespoons raw pumpkin seeds

Sea salt and black pepper

For the Lemon-Dijon Vinaigrette:

3 tablespoons extra virgin olive oil

1 tablespoon fresh lemon juice

1 teaspoon Dijon mustard

1 small garlic clove, minced

Sea salt and black pepper to taste

1. Season the salmon with sea salt and pepper. Grill or bake at 375°F (190°C) for 10–12 minutes, or until just cooked through and flakey. Let cool slightly and break into large chunks.

2. Divide mixed greens into two bowls. Top with avocado slices, cucumber, shredded carrot, pumpkin seeds, and salmon.

3. Whisk together olive oil, lemon juice, Dijon mustard, garlic, salt, and pepper in a small bowl or shake in a jar.

4. Drizzle vinaigrette over each salad, toss lightly, and eat while the salmon is still slightly warm or at room temp.

Optional Add-Ons:

Add fermented sauerkraut for gut support.

Swap pumpkin seeds for walnuts or hemp seeds.

Use canned wild salmon (in water or olive oil) if you're short on time.

Rainbow Slaw

Prep Time: 15 minutes

Servings: 4 (as a side)

Slaw Base:

1 cup shredded red cabbage

1 cup shredded green cabbage

1 large carrot, julienned or shredded

3–4 radishes, thinly sliced or matchsticked

2 green onions, thinly sliced

¼ cup chopped fresh cilantro

Ginger-Lime Slaw Dressing:

Juice of 1–2 limes (about 3 tablespoons)

1 tablespoon rice vinegar

1 tablespoon toasted sesame oil

1 tablespoon coconut aminos (or tamari)

1 tablespoon fresh grated ginger

Pinch of sea salt, to taste

1. In a large mixing bowl, combine all the slaw ingredients—cabbages, carrot, radish, green onion, and cilantro. Toss well.

2. In a small bowl or jar, whisk together lime juice, rice vinegar, sesame oil, coconut aminos, and grated ginger. Taste and adjust lime or salt if needed.

3. Pour the dressing over the slaw and toss until everything's well coated. Let sit for at least 10–15 minutes before serving to let the flavors meld.

4. Serve cold or at room temp. Store leftovers in an airtight container in the fridge for up to 3 days—it just gets better as it sits.

Pro Tip:

Add a handful of chopped cashews or toasted pumpkin seeds for extra crunch and healthy fats, or top with grilled wild salmon or tempeh to make it a full meal.

Warm Quinoa & Roasted Veggie Salad with Garlic-Tahini Dressing

Prep Time: 15 minutes

Cook Time: 30 minutes

Servings: 2–3

Base:

Roasted Veggies:

¾ cup dry quinoa (yields \~2 cups cooked)

1 medium sweet potato, peeled and cubed

1 ½ cups water or broth

1 zucchini, chopped

1 cup fresh arugula

1 red bell pepper, sliced

2 tablespoons hemp seeds

½ red onion, sliced

1 tablespoon extra-virgin olive oil

Garlic-Tahini Dressing:

Sea salt and black pepper, to taste

2 tablespoons tahini

Optional: ½ teaspoon smoked paprika or turmeric

Juice of ½ lemon

1 clove garlic, grated or finely minced

2–3 tablespoons warm water (to thin)

¼ teaspoon ground cumin

Pinch of sea salt

1. Preheat oven to 400°F (200°C). Toss sweet potatoes, zucchini, bell pepper, and red onion with olive oil, salt, pepper, and spices. Spread on a parchment-lined baking sheet. Roast for 25–30 minutes, flipping halfway, until tender and caramelized.

2. Rinse quinoa under cold water. Add to a pot with water or broth. Bring to a boil, then reduce heat, cover, and simmer for 15 minutes. Remove from heat and let sit covered for 5 more minutes. Fluff with a fork.

3. In a small bowl or jar, whisk together tahini, lemon juice, garlic, cumin, and sea salt. Add warm water a bit at a time until smooth and pourable.

4. In bowls, layer warm quinoa, roasted veggies, fresh arugula, and hemp seeds. Drizzle generously with the garlic-tahini dressing.

Batch Tip:

Double the veggies and quinoa to build easy lunches for the week. Store the dressing separately to keep it fresh.

Beet & Walnut Detox Salad

Prep Time: 15 minutes

Cook Time: 30 minutes (if roasting beets)

Servings: 2

Salad:

2 medium beets, roasted or steamed, peeled and sliced

2 cups arugula (or mixed greens)

½ cup crushed walnuts (raw or lightly toasted)

1 orange, peeled and segmented

½ small fennel bulb, thinly sliced (use a mandoline if you have one)

Citrus Vinaigrette:

3 tablespoons fresh orange juice

2 tablespoons extra virgin olive oil

1 tablespoon apple cider vinegar

½ teaspoon Dijon mustard

¼ teaspoon ground turmeric

Pinch of sea salt and black pepper

1. Cook the beets:

Roasting: Wrap beets in foil and roast at 400°F (200°C) for 30–40 minutes until fork-tender.

Steaming: Peel and dice beets, steam for 15–20 minutes. Let cool. (You can also buy pre-cooked beets for shortcuts—just check ingredients.)

2. Whisk together orange juice, olive oil, apple cider vinegar, Dijon, turmeric, salt, and pepper until emulsified.

3. In a large bowl or two serving plates, layer arugula, beet slices, orange segments, fennel, and walnuts.

4. Spoon dressing over the salad right before serving. Toss gently or leave it layered for visual appeal.

Pro Tip:

Add a scoop of cooked quinoa or lentils to turn this into a hearty meal. Keeps well for up to 2 days in the fridge (dressing stored separately).

YOUR BODY DOES NOT HATE YOU, YOU'RE INFLAMED

Curried Chickpea & Kale Crunch Salad

Prep Time: 15 minutes

Cook Time: 25 minutes (for chickpeas)

Servings: 2 large or 3–4 sides

Salad Base:

1 bunch kale, stems removed, leaves torn or chopped

1 tablespoon olive oil

1½ cups cooked chickpeas or 1 can, drained & rinsed

1 teaspoon olive oil (for roasting chickpeas)

½ teaspoon sea salt

1 teaspoon curry powder

½ cup shredded carrots

¼ cup thinly sliced red onion

¼ cup raisins (or chopped dates)

2 tablespoons sunflower seeds (raw or lightly toasted)

Golden Curry Dressing:

2 tablespoons tahini

2 tablespoons extra virgin olive oil

Juice of 1 lemon (about 2 tablespoons)

1 clove garlic, finely minced

½ teaspoon turmeric

1 teaspoon curry powder

Pinch of sea salt

Water to thin (start with 1 tablespoon)

1. Preheat oven to 400°F (200°C). Toss chickpeas with 1 tsp olive oil, curry powder, and sea salt. Spread on a baking sheet and roast for 20–25 minutes, shaking halfway through, until crisp and golden.

2. Add torn kale to a large bowl with 1 tbsp olive oil and a small pinch of salt. Massage with your hands for 2–3 minutes until it softens and darkens in color.

3. In a small bowl or jar, whisk together tahini, olive oil, lemon juice, garlic, turmeric, curry powder, and salt. Add water 1 tsp at a time until desired consistency is reached (creamy but pourable).

4. To the massaged kale, add shredded carrots, red onion, raisins, and sunflower seeds. Pour on the dressing and toss to coat everything evenly.

5. Finish with the roasted chickpeas right before serving to keep them crunchy.

Tip: Make the chickpeas in bulk and store in an airtight container—they're great for snacking or tossing onto any salad.

Avocado, Grapefruit & Arugula Salad with Honey-Mint Citrus Dressing

Prep Time: 10 minutes

Servings: 2

Salad Base:

4 cups fresh arugula, rinsed and dried

1 ripe avocado, sliced or cubed

1 large grapefruit, peeled and segmented (membranes removed)

2 tablespoons slivered almonds (lightly toasted, optional)

Dressing:

2 tablespoons fresh grapefruit juice (squeezed from segmented grapefruit)

2 tablespoons extra virgin olive oil

1 teaspoon raw honey or date syrup

1 tablespoon finely chopped fresh mint

Pinch of sea salt

1. In a small bowl or jar, whisk together grapefruit juice, olive oil, honey (if using), mint, and sea salt until emulsified.

2. In a large bowl, combine arugula, avocado, and grapefruit segments. Gently toss to mix.

3. Sprinkle with slivered almonds. Drizzle with dressing just before serving.

4. This salad is best enjoyed fresh—bright, light, and satisfying.

Sardine & Olive Protein Salad

Prep Time: 10 minutes

Servings: 2

1 large head romaine lettuce, chopped

1 can (3.75 oz) wild-caught sardines in olive oil or water, drained

1 cup cherry tomatoes, halved

½ cucumber, chopped

¼ cup pitted Kalamata or green olives, sliced

2 tablespoons chopped fresh parsley

Simple Lemon-Olive Oil Dressing:

Juice of 1 lemon (about 2 tablespoons)

3 tablespoons extra virgin olive oil

1 tablespoon caper brine (or white wine vinegar)

Freshly ground black pepper, to taste

Optional: pinch of sea salt or minced garlic

1. Whisk together lemon juice, olive oil, caper brine, and black pepper in a small bowl or shake in a jar.

2. In a large bowl, combine chopped romaine, cherry tomatoes, cucumber, olives, and parsley.

3. Gently break the sardines into bite-sized chunks and scatter over the top. Don't overmix—they're delicate.

4. Drizzle the dressing over the salad and toss gently until everything is lightly coated.

5. This is best fresh, but leftovers keep in the fridge (undressed) for up to 1 day.

Pro Tip:

If you're new to sardines, start with skinless & boneless options packed in olive oil—they're milder and easier to love. You can also sub in mackerel or wild salmon for variety.

Roasted Broccoli & Tahini Salad

Prep Time: 10 minutes

Cook Time: 20 minutes

Servings: 2

Salad Base:

1 small head of broccoli, cut into florets

1 tablespoon olive oil

Sea salt and black pepper to taste

3 cups mixed greens (arugula, spinach, or spring mix)

¼ red onion, thinly sliced

¼ cup pomegranate seeds

1 tablespoon hemp hearts

Zesty Tahini Dressing:

2 tablespoons tahini

1 tablespoon fresh lemon juice

1 garlic clove, minced

2–3 tablespoons water

¼ teaspoon ground cumin

Pinch of cayenne

Sea salt to taste

1. Preheat oven to 400°F (200°C). Toss broccoli florets in olive oil, salt, and pepper. Roast on a lined baking sheet for 20 minutes, turning halfway, until crisp-tender and golden on the edges.

2. In a small bowl or jar, whisk together tahini, lemon juice, garlic, cumin, cayenne, and a pinch of salt. Add water gradually until the dressing is creamy and pourable.

3. In a large bowl or two serving bowls, layer mixed greens, roasted broccoli, red onion, and pomegranate seeds. Drizzle with tahini dressing.

4. Sprinkle with hemp hearts just before serving for a nutty crunch and added omega-3s.

Pro Tip:

Make extra broccoli and dressing—you'll want to use them again tomorrow. Both keep well in the fridge for 3–4 days. Great for meal prep.

YOUR BODY DOES NOT HATE YOU, YOU'RE INFLAMED

Gut-Healing Fermented Veggie Salad

Prep Time: 10 minutes

Servings: 2

Salad Base:

4 cups mixed leafy greens (arugula, spinach, romaine)

½ cup fermented carrots or raw sauerkraut (look for raw or unpasteurized on the label)

½ ripe avocado, sliced or cubed

1 cup shredded cooked chicken or cubed organic tofu (lightly pan-seared or steamed)

1 small zucchini, grated or spiralized

Optional toppings: sprinkle of hemp seeds, sesame seeds, or nori flakes

Miso-Ginger Dressing:

1 tablespoon unpasteurized miso paste (white or yellow for a mellow flavor)

1 teaspoon fresh grated ginger

1 tablespoon apple cider vinegar (with the mother)

1 teaspoon toasted sesame oil

2–3 tablespoons water

1. In a small bowl or jar, whisk together miso, ginger, apple cider vinegar, and sesame oil. Add water gradually until smooth and pourable.

2. In a large bowl, combine mixed greens, fermented veggies, avocado, zucchini, and your choice of protein.

3. Drizzle dressing over the salad, toss gently, and taste for salt (miso is salty, so you likely won't need more).

4. Top with seeds or nori if using, and enjoy while the greens are still fresh and crisp.

This one's great for meal-prep too—just store the dressing separately until ready to eat.

DESSERTS & SWEET TREATS

- Ditch refined sugar—opt for raw honey, maple syrup, dates, or monk fruit (in moderation).
- Use real ingredients—coconut flour, almond flour, cacao, spices, nuts, seeds.
- Portion matters. Even anti-inflammatory sweets can become sugar bombs if you overdo them.
- Batch prep a couple treats each week to avoid last-minute junk cravings.

Golden Milk Chia Pudding

Prep Time: 5 minutes

Soak Time: Overnight (or at least 4 hours)

Servings: 2

½ cup chia seeds

2 cups full-fat coconut milk

¾ teaspoon ground turmeric

½ teaspoon ground cinnamon

¼ teaspoon ground ginger

⅛ teaspoon ground black pepper

1 teaspoon pure vanilla extract

1–2 teaspoons raw honey or monk fruit sweetener

Pinch of sea salt

Optional Toppings:

Crushed pistachios (unsalted)

Fresh berries (blueberries, raspberries, or pomegranate seeds)

Sprinkle of extra cinnamon

1. In a medium bowl or jar, whisk together coconut milk, turmeric, cinnamon, ginger, black pepper, vanilla, sweetener, and salt.

2. Stir in the chia seeds and mix well to avoid clumps. Let sit for 10 minutes, then stir again to redistribute.

3. Cover and refrigerate overnight (or for at least 4 hours) until thick and pudding-like.

4. Give it a quick stir, then divide into two bowls or jars. Top with crushed pistachios and berries, and dust with extra cinnamon if desired.

Dark Chocolate Avocado Mousse

Prep Time: 5 minutes

Chill Time: 30 minutes (optional, for best texture)

Servings: 2

1 ripe avocado (make sure it's soft and green inside)

3 tablespoons raw cacao powder (not Dutch-processed cocoa)

2–3 tablespoons pure maple syrup

½ teaspoon vanilla extract

Pinch of sea salt

Optional:

1 tablespoon almond butter

¼ teaspoon ground cinnamon

Splash of non-dairy milk if needed for blending

1. Scoop avocado into a blender or food processor. Add cacao, maple syrup, vanilla, sea salt, and any optional add-ins.

2. Blend until silky, scraping down sides as needed. If too thick, add 1–2 teaspoons of almond milk at a time until mousse consistency forms.

3. Scoop into ramekins or small bowls. Chill in the fridge for 30 minutes for a thicker, pudding-like texture—or enjoy it immediately if you're impatient (no judgment).

4. Top with a few crushed walnuts, cacao nibs, or a sprinkle of cinnamon if you're feeling fancy.

Berry Coconut Crumble

Prep Time: 10 minutes

Cook Time: 25–30 minutes

Servings: 4

For the filling:

3 cups mixed berries (fresh or frozen—blueberries, raspberries, blackberries)

1 tablespoon arrowroot powder or tapioca starch

1–2 teaspoons raw honey or maple syrup

½ teaspoon vanilla extract

Pinch of sea salt

For the crumble topping:

¾ cup almond flour

½ cup unsweetened shredded coconut

1 teaspoon ground cinnamon

3 tablespoons coconut oil (solid or softened)

1 tablespoon maple syrup or raw honey

Pinch of sea salt

1. Set your oven to 350°F (175°C). Lightly grease a small baking dish with coconut oil.

2. In a bowl, toss the berries with arrowroot, vanilla, sea salt, and sweetener if using. Pour into the baking dish and spread evenly.

3. In another bowl, mix almond flour, shredded coconut, cinnamon, and sea salt. Add coconut oil and sweetener. Use a fork or your fingers to blend until crumbly and moist.

4. Sprinkle the crumble mixture evenly over the berries.

5. Bake for 25–30 minutes until the topping is golden and the berries are bubbling at the edges.

6. Let sit for 5–10 minutes before serving. Enjoy warm as is, or top with a dollop of coconut yogurt or chia pudding.

Pro Tip:

This keeps well in the fridge for 3–4 days and reheats nicely. You can also use this crumble topping on baked apples or pears for variety.

No-Bake Turmeric Ginger Bites

Prep Time: 10 minutes

Chill Time: 20–30 minutes

Servings: 10–12 bites

1 cup almond flour

1 tablespoon ground turmeric

1 teaspoon ground ginger

½ teaspoon ground cinnamon

2 tablespoons coconut oil (melted)

1½ tablespoons pure maple syrup (or raw honey)

½ teaspoon pure vanilla extract

Pinch of sea salt

Optional: 1–2 teaspoons water if mixture is too dry

Coating: shredded coconut or hemp seeds for rolling

1. In a medium bowl, whisk together almond flour, turmeric, ginger, cinnamon, and sea salt.

2. Stir in melted coconut oil, maple syrup, and vanilla. Mix until a dough forms. If it feels too crumbly, add water 1 tsp at a time.

3. Scoop out heaping teaspoons of the mixture and roll into bite-sized balls.

4. Roll each ball in shredded coconut or hemp seeds until coated.

5. Place bites in the fridge for 20–30 minutes to firm up, or eat them soft right away.

6. Keep in an airtight container in the fridge for up to a week, or freeze for longer.

Pro Tip: These are great for curbing sugar cravings at night without spiking inflammation.

Baked Apples with Walnuts & Cinnamon

Prep Time: 10 minutes

Cook Time: 30–35 minutes

Servings: 2 (easily doubled)

2 medium organic apples (Honeycrisp, Pink Lady, or Fuji work great)

¼ cup chopped raw walnuts

2 tablespoons raisins (unsweetened)

1 teaspoon ground cinnamon

1 tablespoon coconut oil or ghee (melted)

Optional: pinch of sea salt, dash of nutmeg or ground ginger

Optional: drizzle of raw honey or date syrup (1 tsp total)

1. Set to 350°F (175°C).

2. Wash and core the apples, leaving the bottom intact to create a natural bowl.

3. In a small bowl, mix walnuts, raisins, cinnamon, and melted coconut oil or ghee. Add optional pinch of salt or extra spice if desired.

4. Fill the cored centers with the mixture, pressing down gently to pack.

5. Place apples in a small baking dish. Add 1–2 tablespoons water to the bottom of the dish to keep them moist. Cover loosely with foil and bake for 20 minutes. Remove foil and bake another 10–15 minutes until apples are soft and golden.

6. Optional drizzle of raw honey or date syrup before serving. Great as dessert, snack, or even breakfast.

Matcha Coconut Fat Bombs

Prep Time: 10 minutes

Chill Time: 30–60 minutes

Servings: 10–12 fat bombs

½ cup coconut butter (softened)

¼ cup coconut oil

1½ teaspoons matcha powder (ceremonial grade if possible)

1 teaspoon vanilla extract

⅛ teaspoon fine sea salt

1–2 teaspoons monk fruit sweetener or stevia

1. In a small saucepan over low heat (or in a double boiler), gently melt coconut butter and coconut oil together. Stir continuously to avoid burning.

2. Once melted, remove from heat. Stir in matcha, vanilla, salt, and sweetener. Whisk until completely smooth.

3. Let the mixture cool slightly (so it's easier to handle but not solid). Scoop into small silicone molds or form into balls using a small cookie scoop or spoon.

4. Place in the fridge or freezer for 30–60 minutes until firm.

5. Keep refrigerated in an airtight container for up to 2 weeks—or freeze for longer shelf life.

Pro Tip:

Add 1 tbsp of collagen peptides or hemp protein to boost the protein content. Want a chocolate variation? Sub 1 tsp of matcha with 1 tbsp raw cacao powder.

YOUR BODY DOES NOT HATE YOU, YOU'RE INFLAMED

Frozen Banana-Nut Bark

Prep Time: 10 minutes

Freeze Time: 1–2 hours

Servings: About 6–8 small pieces

2 ripe (but firm) bananas, sliced into ¼-inch rounds

2 tablespoons almond butter or tahini (unsweetened, no additives)

¼ cup chopped walnuts or pecans

¼ cup dark chocolate chips or chunks (85% cacao or higher)

½ teaspoon coconut oil

Optional: pinch of sea salt, sprinkle of cinnamon

1. Line a baking sheet or plate with parchment paper.

2. Arrange banana slices in a single layer. You can place them close together to form a bark "sheet" or spaced out for individual bites.

3. Dollop a little almond butter or tahini onto each banana slice and gently spread it with the back of a spoon.

4. Sprinkle chopped walnuts or pecans evenly over the top.

5. Melt the dark chocolate with coconut oil in a small pan over low heat or microwave in 15-second bursts, stirring between. Drizzle generously over the bananas.

6. Pop the tray into the freezer for 1–2 hours or until firm.

7. Once frozen, break into bark-style pieces or keep the slices as-is. Store in a freezer-safe container for up to 2 weeks..

Coconut Yogurt Parfait

Prep Time: 5 minutes

Servings: 1

1 cup unsweetened coconut yogurt (look for clean brands with live cultures, no added sugars)

½ cup fresh or frozen organic berries (blueberries, raspberries, or strawberries)

1 tablespoon hemp seeds

¼ teaspoon ground cinnamon

Optional: ¼ cup grain-free granola (check for clean ingredients: nuts, seeds, coconut, spices)

1. Spoon half the coconut yogurt into a bowl or jar.

2. Layer in half of the berries, sprinkle with some cinnamon and half the hemp seeds.

3. Add remaining yogurt, top with more berries, the rest of the hemp seeds, and another dusting of cinnamon.

4. Add grain-free granola on top just before eating to keep it crunchy.

Tips:

Great as a quick breakfast, snack, or even a light dessert.

Swap hemp seeds for ground flax or chia for variety.

Add a drizzle of raw honey or date syrup if you need a little extra sweetness.

Sweet Potato Brownie Bites

Prep Time: 10 minutes

Cook Time: 20–25 minutes

Servings: 12 mini brownie bites

1 cup mashed cooked sweet potato (about 1 medium sweet potato)

½ cup almond flour

¼ cup unsweetened cacao powder (not cocoa—go raw if possible)

¼ cup pure maple syrup

1 egg or flax egg (1 tbsp ground flax + 2.5 tbsp water, mixed and set for 5 min)

1 teaspoon vanilla extract

¼ teaspoon sea salt

Optional:

2 tablespoons mini dark chocolate chips (70%+ cacao, no dairy or soy)

Chopped walnuts or pecans for topping

1. Set to 350°F (175°C). Lightly grease a mini muffin tin or use silicone liners.

2. In a bowl, combine mashed sweet potato, maple syrup, egg/flax egg, and vanilla. Stir until smooth.

3. Mix in almond flour, cacao powder, and salt. Stir until fully combined. Fold in chocolate chips if using.

4. Spoon batter into mini muffin cups, filling each about ¾ full. Top with chopped nuts if desired.

5. Bake for 20–25 minutes, or until set and a toothpick comes out with a few moist crumbs.

6. Let cool for 10–15 minutes before removing from pan. They'll firm up as they cool.

Storage Tip:

Keep in the fridge for up to 5 days, or freeze for longer. Great as a pre-workout bite or clean dessert.

Spiced Quinoa Porridge with Apple & Nuts

Prep Time: 5 minutes

Cook Time: 15 minutes

Servings: 2

1 cup cooked quinoa (or ½ cup uncooked, rinsed well)

1 cup unsweetened almond milk (plus more to thin, if needed)

1 small apple, grated (with skin on for fiber)

½ teaspoon ground cinnamon

⅛ teaspoon ground nutmeg

Pinch of sea salt

1 teaspoon pure maple syrup or raw honey

Toppings (per serving):

2 tablespoons chopped walnuts

1 tablespoon hemp hearts

Drizzle of almond butter (1 teaspoon or to taste)

Optional: extra cinnamon, apple slices, or chia seeds

1. Rinse ½ cup quinoa under cold water. In a small pot, combine with 1 cup water. Bring to a boil, then cover and simmer for 12–15 minutes until fluffy. Let sit covered for 5 minutes, then fluff with a fork.

2. In a saucepan, combine 1 cup cooked quinoa with almond milk, grated apple, cinnamon, nutmeg, and salt. Simmer over low heat for 5–7 minutes until warm, thickened, and creamy. Stir occasionally and add more almond milk as needed.

3. Stir in maple syrup or honey if using. Adjust spices to taste.

4. Pour into bowls. Top each with walnuts, hemp hearts, and a drizzle of almond butter. Add extra apple slices or spices if desired.

TEAS & DRINKS

- Avoid sweeteners and artificial flavors. Even natural flavors can mess with your gut and brain.
- Choose organic loose leaf or fresh herbs when possible.
- Keep an herbal tea station or make big batches of iced versions to sip through the day.

Timing matters:

- Morning: green tea or ginger-lemon
- Midday: matcha or hibiscus
- Evening: rooibos, tulsi, or golden milk

Turmeric Ginger Tea (Golden Elixir)

Prep Time: 5 minutes

Cook Time: 10–15 minutes simmer time

Servings: 2

1½ cups water

1-inch piece fresh turmeric root, peeled and sliced

1-inch piece fresh ginger root, peeled and sliced

¼ teaspoon ground cinnamon (or 1 small stick)

1 pinch freshly ground black pepper

Juice of ½ lemon

Optional:

1 teaspoon raw honey (added after steeping)

½ teaspoon coconut oil

1. In a small saucepan, bring water to a boil. Add turmeric, ginger, cinnamon, and black pepper. Lower the heat and simmer gently for 10–15 minutes.

2. Remove from heat. Strain into a mug. Stir in lemon juice and, if using, add a small amount of raw honey or coconut oil.

3. Sip slowly. It's especially good on an empty stomach in the morning or post-meal to support digestion.

Pro Tip:

Make a batch in advance and store in the fridge for up to 3 days. Reheat gently or serve chilled over ice for a refreshing twist.

Green Tea (Unflavored, Organic)

Prep Time: 2 minutes

Steep Time: 2–5 minutes

Servings: 1

1 teaspoon loose-leaf organic green tea (or 1 unflavored, organic green tea bag—matcha, sencha, or jasmine)*

1 cup hot water (not boiling, about 160–180°F / 70–80°C)

1 lemon wedge

1. Avoid boiling—green tea gets bitter if the water's too hot. Aim for just-steaming water.

2. Place tea leaves or bag in a mug. Pour over hot water and steep for 2–3 minutes for a mild brew, up to 5 minutes for more intensity. Remove leaves or bag.

3. Squeeze in a little lemon for extra vitamin C and enhanced polyphenol absorption.

4. Ideal as a mid-morning or early afternoon anti-inflammatory ritual. Avoid adding sweeteners—this tea is about clean, medicinal support.

Tip:

If using matcha, whisk ½ tsp matcha powder into warm water instead of steeping. You're drinking the whole leaf, so it's stronger—start small.

Holy Basil (Tulsi) Tea

Prep Time: 2 minutes

Brew Time: 5–10 minutes

Servings: 1

1 tsp dried holy basil leaves or 1 Tulsi tea bag (Fresh tulsi leaves work too—use 4–5 per cup, lightly crushed)*

1 cup hot water (just off the boil)

Optional additions:

1–2 thin slices fresh ginger

1 small cinnamon stick or pinch of ground cinnamon

Splash of unsweetened nut milk

1. Heat water to just below a rolling boil (around 200°F / 93°C).

2. Pour hot water over the tulsi leaves or tea bag. Add ginger or cinnamon if using. Cover and steep for 5–10 minutes.

3. Remove the tea bag or strain out loose leaves and add-ins. Add a splash of nut milk if desired. Sip slowly, ideally away from meals.

Ginger-Lemon Infusion

Prep Time: 5 minutes

Cook Time: 10 minutes (steeping)

Servings: 1 mug (can be scaled up)

1–2 inches fresh ginger root, sliced thin or grated

Juice of ½ fresh lemon

1½ cups hot water (just below boiling)

Optional: pinch of cayenne pepper

1. Slice or grate the ginger. Grated gives a stronger, more intense flavor and extraction.

2. Add ginger to a mug or teapot and pour hot water over it. Let steep for 8–10 minutes covered.

3. Once steeped, stir in the fresh lemon juice and a pinch of cayenne if you like a spicy edge.

4. Strain if desired and enjoy warm. Drink slowly, ideally on an empty stomach in the morning or after meals to aid digestion.

Hibiscus Tea (Chilled or Hot)

Prep Time: 5 minutes

Brew Time: 10–15 minutes

Servings: 2

2 tablespoons dried hibiscus petals (also called roselle or flor de Jamaica)

2½ cups hot water (just off the boil)

1 cinnamon stick

1–2 slices of fresh orange (with peel)

Optional: 1–2 teaspoons raw honey or a few drops of stevia (added after brewing, once cooled slightly)

For Hot Tea:

1. Place hibiscus petals, cinnamon stick, and orange slices into a teapot or heatproof jar. Pour in hot water.

2. Let it sit for 10–15 minutes, covered to retain the essential oils.

3. Strain out solids. Add raw honey if desired, but wait until it cools slightly to preserve enzymes.

For Iced Tea:

1. Follow the steps above, then...

2. Let cool to room temp, then transfer to the fridge for at least 1 hour.

3. Garnish with an extra orange slice or a few fresh mint leaves if you're feeling fancy.

Cinnamon Rooibos Latte

Prep Time: 5 minutes

Cook Time: 5 minutes

Servings: 1

1 rooibos tea bag or 1 tbsp loose-leaf rooibos

1 cup hot water

½ cup unsweetened almond milk or coconut milk

¼ teaspoon ground cinnamon

¼ teaspoon pure vanilla extract

Optional: 1 tsp raw honey or date syrup (if desired)

1. Steep the rooibos tea in 1 cup of hot water for at least 5 minutes (longer for stronger flavor).

2. While the tea brews, warm the almond or coconut milk in a small pot over low heat. Whisk in cinnamon and vanilla. (Use a milk frother or immersion blender if you want it foamy.)

3. Remove tea bag or strain leaves. Pour the spiced milk into your mug with the brewed rooibos tea.

4. Add raw honey or date syrup if using, stir, and sprinkle a pinch of cinnamon on top. Sip warm.

Green Juice (No Fruit Bombs)

Prep Time: 10 minutes

Juicing Time: 5 minutes

Servings: 2 small or 1 large

1 large cucumber (peeled if waxy)

3–4 celery stalks

1 cup kale leaves (stems removed) or spinach

½ bunch fresh parsley

1-inch piece of fresh ginger (peeled)

½ lemon, peeled

Optional add-ins:

1-inch piece fresh turmeric root (or ¼ tsp ground)

A few fresh mint leaves

1. Wash and prep all ingredients.

2. Run everything through a juicer, starting with softer ingredients (parsley, kale), then cucumber and celery to flush it through.

3. Stir and serve immediately. You can also chill it for 10–15 minutes if you like it cold.

(Blender Version):

1. Chop ingredients into smaller chunks.

2. Add all ingredients to a high-speed blender with ½ to 1 cup cold filtered water.

3. Blend until smooth, then strain through a fine mesh strainer, nut milk bag, or cheesecloth to remove pulp.

4. Pour and serve.

Pro Tip: Drink this on an empty stomach in the morning or between meals for maximum absorption and digestive benefits.

YOUR BODY DOES NOT HATE YOU, YOU'RE INFLAMED

Bone Broth Elixir

Prep Time: 5 minutes

Simmer Time (if making broth from scratch): 12–24 hours

Serving Size: 1 mug (recipe easily scales up)

1 cup high-quality bone broth (chicken or beef) — homemade or store-bought (look for organic, no additives)

¼ teaspoon ground turmeric

Pinch of freshly ground black pepper (enhances curcumin absorption)

¼ teaspoon grated fresh ginger (or ⅛ tsp ground ginger)

1 teaspoon fresh lemon juice

Optional:

Pinch of sea salt

1 scoop collagen peptides (unflavored)

1. In a small saucepan, gently warm the bone broth over low to medium heat until hot but not boiling.

2. Stir in turmeric, black pepper, ginger, and lemon juice. If using collagen powder, whisk it in thoroughly until dissolved.

3. Add a pinch of sea salt if desired. Pour into a mug and sip slowly.

Pro Tip:

Make a big batch of broth and freeze it in single-serve portions. Reheat and add the elixir ingredients when needed—perfect for mornings, cold days, or when your gut needs a reset.

Matcha Coconut Latte

Prep Time: 5 minutes

Cook Time: 3–5 minutes

Servings: 1

1 teaspoon ceremonial-grade matcha powder

2 tablespoons hot (but not boiling) water

¾ cup steamed coconut milk

¼ teaspoon pure vanilla extract

Pinch of ground cinnamon

Optional: ½ teaspoon raw honey or a couple drops
of monk fruit for sweetness

1. In a mug or bowl, whisk matcha powder with hot water using a bamboo whisk or milk frother until smooth and frothy. No clumps allowed.

2. Warm the coconut milk in a small saucepan over medium heat until hot but not boiling. Froth with a hand frother if desired.

3. Pour the steamed coconut milk into your matcha. Stir in vanilla, cinnamon, and sweetener if using.

4. Enjoy slowly—this is a calm energy drink, not a shot of espresso.

KID-FRIENDLY

O
P
T
I
ONS

- Keep it colorful and fun—skewers, cut shapes, dips, or build-your-own meals.
- Let them help prep—ownership = fewer complaints.
- Use familiar foods with upgraded ingredients (e.g., grain-free pancakes, real fruit popsicles).
- Watch out for kid marketing on packaged foods—it usually means extra sugar, seed oils, or junk.

Sweet Potato Fries with Avocado Dip

Prep Time: 10 minutes

Cook Time: 25–30 minutes

Serving Size: Serves 2–3 kids

For the Fries:

1 large sweet potato, peeled and cut into wedges or sticks

1 tablespoon olive oil

¼ teaspoon ground cinnamon

Pinch of sea salt

For the Avocado Dip:

1 ripe avocado

1 tablespoon fresh lime juice

Pinch of garlic powder or ¼ small garlic clove (grated)

Pinch of sea salt

1. Preheat oven to 400°F (200°C). Toss sweet potato wedges with olive oil, cinnamon, and sea salt.

2. Spread fries on a parchment-lined baking sheet in a single layer. Bake for 25–30 minutes, flipping halfway, until golden and tender with crisp edges.

3. In a small bowl, mash the avocado with lime juice, garlic, and salt until smooth and creamy.

4. Let fries cool slightly before serving with the dip on the side for dunking fun.

Pro Tip:

Cut fries into fun shapes or thinner sticks for tiny hands. Leftover dip also works great as a sandwich spread or taco topper.

Turkey & Veggie Meatballs

Prep Time: 15 minutes

Cook Time: 20–25 minutes

Yield: About 18 mini meatballs (serves 3–4 kids)

1 lb ground turkey (preferably organic or pasture-raised)

½ cup grated zucchini (squeezed dry)

½ cup finely grated carrot

¼ cup almond flour

1 garlic clove, minced (or ¼ teaspoon garlic powder)

½ teaspoon dried oregano or Italian herbs

¼ teaspoon sea salt

Optional: 1 egg (helps bind, but not necessary for small meatballs)

To serve:

Homemade marinara or dairy-free pesto (see earlier recipes)

1. Set oven to 375°F (190°C). Line a baking sheet with parchment paper.

2. In a bowl, combine ground turkey, grated veggies, almond flour, garlic, herbs, and salt. Mix until just combined—don't overwork.

3. Roll mixture into small, kid-sized meatballs and place on baking sheet. Bake for 20–25 minutes, flipping halfway, until golden and cooked through.

4. Let cool slightly before serving with a side of marinara or pesto for dipping fun.

Pro Tip:

Make a double batch and freeze the extras. These meatballs are great in lunchboxes, pasta bowls, or wrapped in lettuce cups.

Rainbow Smoothie Popsicles

Prep Time: 10 minutes

Freeze Time: 4–6 hours

Yield: About 6 popsicles (depending on mold size)

1 ripe banana

½ cup mixed berries (strawberries, blueberries, raspberries) — fresh or frozen

½ cup fresh spinach

1 tablespoon chia seeds

1 cup full-fat canned coconut milk (or unsweetened almond milk)

Optional:

1–2 teaspoons maple syrup or raw honey

1. In a blender, combine banana, berries, chia seeds, and coconut milk. Blend until smooth. For a "rainbow" effect, blend in stages—separate into batches and add spinach to one for a green layer.

2. Pour into popsicle molds in layers (or swirl gently for a marbled look). Tap molds lightly to remove air bubbles.

3. Insert sticks and freeze for 4–6 hours, or until fully set.

4. Run molds briefly under warm water to release popsicles.

Pro Tip:

Add a few fresh fruit chunks to the molds before pouring in the smoothie for a fun surprise in every bite. Great for teething toddlers or a cool afternoon treat!

Cauliflower Tater Tots

Prep Time: 15 minutes

Cook Time: 25–30 minutes (bake) or 15 minutes (air fryer)

Yield: About 20 tots

2 cups cauliflower florets (steamed until tender, then cooled)

¼ cup almond flour

1 egg

1 small garlic clove, minced (or ¼ tsp garlic powder)

1 tablespoon nutritional yeast (for cheesy flavor)

¼ teaspoon sea salt

Optional:

Pinch of dried herbs (like parsley or oregano)

Olive oil spray

1. Preheat oven or air fryer:

Oven: 400°F (200°C). Line a baking sheet with parchment paper.

Air fryer: Preheat to 375°F (190°C).

2. In a food processor, pulse the steamed cauliflower until finely chopped (not pureed). Transfer to a bowl and mix with almond flour, egg, garlic, nutritional yeast, salt, and herbs (if using).

3. Scoop about 1 tablespoon of mixture and shape into mini tot shapes using your hands.

4. Bake or air-fry:

Oven: Place tots on baking sheet, spray lightly with olive oil, and bake for 25–30 minutes, flipping halfway.

Air fryer: Place in basket, spray with oil, and cook for about 15 minutes, shaking halfway through, until golden and crisp.

Pro Tip:

Serve with a side of homemade ketchup or dairy-free ranch for dunking. Great for lunchboxes or snack time!

DIY Lunchbox Bento

Prep Time: 10 minutes

Total Time: 10 minutes

Yield: 1 kid-sized bento box (easily scaled up)

3–4 slices of nitrate-free turkey or chicken (roll-ups or bite-sized pieces)

½ cup sliced cucumbers, carrots, or bell peppers

½ cup fresh berries or apple slices (tossed in lemon juice to prevent browning)

2–3 tablespoons hummus or a nut-free veggie dip (like garlic-herb dip)

Small handful of olives or unsalted nuts (omit or swap for seeds if under age 4)

Optional Add-Ins:

Hard-boiled egg

Grain-free crackers

A square of dark chocolate (70%+, dairy-free)

1. In a lunchbox with compartments or small containers, arrange the protein, veggies, fruit, dip, and sides.

2. Keep cold with an ice pack if sending to school. Use silicone muffin cups to divide and keep items separate and fun.

Pro Tip:

Let kids help pick their components—it builds independence and boosts the chance they'll eat it all! Rotate in new veggies or dips weekly to keep it exciting.

YOUR BODY DOES NOT HATE YOU, YOU'RE INFLAMED

Zucchini & Banana Mini Muffins

Prep Time: 10 minutes

Bake Time: 15–18 minutes

Yield: 12 mini muffins

1 ripe banana, mashed

½ cup finely grated zucchini (squeezed to remove excess moisture)

1 cup almond flour

1 egg or flax egg (1 tbsp ground flax + 3 tbsp water, rested 5 min)

1½ teaspoons cinnamon

1 tablespoon pure maple syrup

½ teaspoon baking soda

½ teaspoon vanilla extract

Pinch of sea salt

Optional:

Mini dairy-free chocolate chips or chopped walnuts (if age-appropriate)

1. Set to 350°F (175°C). Line a mini muffin tin with paper liners or grease lightly with coconut oil.

2. In a bowl, whisk together mashed banana, zucchini, egg/flax egg, maple syrup, and vanilla. Add almond flour, cinnamon, baking soda, and salt. Stir until just combined.

3. Divide batter evenly among muffin cups. Bake for 15–18 minutes, or until tops are golden and a toothpick comes out clean.

4. Let cool in pan for a few minutes before transferring to a wire rack.

Pro Tip:

Freeze extras for quick grab-and-go snacks. These muffins are soft, moist, and perfect for breakfast or lunchboxes—especially for picky eaters!

Berry Chia Jam with Almond Butter Roll-Ups

Prep Time: 10 minutes

Chill Time (for jam): 20–30 minutes

Yield: 2 roll-ups (easily scaled)

For the Chia Jam:

1 cup fresh or frozen mixed berries (strawberries, blueberries, raspberries)

1 tablespoon chia seeds

1 teaspoon fresh lemon juice

Optional: ½–1 teaspoon maple syrup

For the Roll-Ups:

2 almond flour tortillas

2 tablespoons almond butter or sunflower seed butter (nut-free option)

2–3 tablespoons prepared berry chia jam

1. In a small saucepan over medium heat, warm the berries until they begin to break down (about 5 minutes). Mash with a fork or potato masher. Stir in chia seeds, lemon juice, and maple syrup if using. Let sit for 20–30 minutes to thicken (or refrigerate to speed it up).

2. Spread almond butter evenly over each tortilla. Top with a layer of chia jam. Roll up tightly.

3. Cut into pinwheels or leave whole for older kids.

Pro Tip:

Make a batch of jam ahead of time—it keeps for up to 1 week in the fridge. Great for toast, yogurt bowls, or overnight oats too!

Chicken Veggie Nuggets

Prep Time: 15 minutes

Cook Time: 20–25 minutes (bake) or 12–15 minutes (air fryer)

Yield: About 15 nuggets

1 lb ground chicken (organic or pasture-raised if possible)

½ cup finely grated zucchini (squeezed dry)

½ cup finely grated carrot

1 small garlic clove, minced (or ¼ tsp garlic powder)

½ teaspoon dried Italian herbs or oregano

½ teaspoon sea salt

¼ cup almond flour (mixed in)

½ cup almond flour (for coating)

Optional: 1 egg

To cook:

Olive oil spray (for crispiness)

1. Preheat oven or air fryer:

Oven: 400°F (200°C). Line a baking sheet with parchment paper.

Air fryer: Preheat to 375°F (190°C).

2. In a large bowl, combine ground chicken, veggies, garlic, herbs, salt, and ¼ cup almond flour. Add egg if using. Mix gently until just combined.

3. Form mixture into small nugget shapes. Roll each in the remaining almond flour to coat.

4. Bake or air-fry:

Oven: Arrange on baking sheet, spray lightly with olive oil, and bake for 20–25 minutes, flipping halfway

Air fryer: Cook for 12–15 minutes, shaking halfway through, until golden and cooked through.

Pro Tip:

Serve with a kid-friendly dipping sauce like beet hummus, guacamole, or golden mustard. Freeze extras for quick lunchbox options or busy weeknights.

Apple Nachos

Prep Time: 5 minutes

Total Time: 5 minutes

Serving Size: 1–2 kids (easily scaled)

1 crisp apple (like Honeycrisp or Fuji), thinly sliced

1–2 tablespoons almond butter (or sunflower seed butter for nut-free option)

1 teaspoon hemp seeds

¼ teaspoon ground cinnamon

1 tablespoon dairy-free dark chocolate chips (mini chips work best)

Optional:

Unsweetened shredded coconut

A light drizzle of raw honey or maple syrup

1. Core and slice the apple into thin wedges. Arrange in a fan or pile on a small plate.

2. Warm the almond butter slightly if needed, then drizzle over the apple slices. Sprinkle with hemp seeds, cinnamon, and chocolate chips. Add any optional toppings.

3. Best enjoyed fresh so the apples stay crisp.

Pro Tip:

Let kids build their own apple nachos with a topping bar for snack time or playdates. It's hands-on and gives them a sense of choice while keeping things healthy.

Coconut Yogurt Parfait Jars

Prep Time: 5 minutes

Total Time: 5 minutes

Yield: 1 jar (easily scaled for batch prep)

½ cup unsweetened coconut yogurt (look for live cultures and no added sugars)

¼ cup fresh berries (blueberries, strawberries, raspberries)

¼ cup grain-free granola (store-bought or homemade)

1 teaspoon raw honey or pure maple syrup

Optional Add-Ins:

Chia seeds or hemp seeds

A dash of cinnamon

Sliced banana or kiwi

1. In a small mason jar or cup, spoon in a layer of coconut yogurt, followed by berries, then granola. Repeat layers if space allows.

2. Top with a light drizzle of raw honey or maple syrup. Add optional seeds or spices as desired.

3. Enjoy right away for crunch, or refrigerate for up to 12 hours if packing for school or snack prep.

Pro Tip:

Let kids assemble their own parfaits—it's a great way to encourage healthy choices and make probiotics feel like a treat!

APPENDIX

Ready-to-Eat Meals From Stores and Great Brands you Can Trust

When selecting prepared meals, prioritize options with whole food ingredients, minimal additives, and healthy fats.

- [Healthy Choice Top Chef Ravioli & Chicken Marinara]
  A balanced meal featuring lean protein and whole grains.

- [Healthy Choice Café Steamers, Chicken Margherita with Balsamic]
  Offers a mix of vegetables and lean protein with a flavorful balsamic sauce.

- [Keto Broccoli Bake Chicken]
  A low-carb option rich in cruciferous vegetables and lean chicken.

Snacks

Choose snacks that are minimally processed, free from added sugars, and rich in fiber and healthy fats.

- [Anti-Inflammatory Snacks and Appetizers]
  A selection designed to combat inflammation during snack times.

- [Bubbies Mochi Triple Chocolate Mochi Ice Cream]
  While a treat, it's made with quality ingredients and can be enjoyed in moderation.

Pantry Staples

Stock your pantry with items that serve as the foundation for anti-inflammatory meals.

- [Organic Extra Virgin Olive Oil Cold Pressed - 2L]
  Rich in monounsaturated fats and antioxidants, it's a staple for cooking and dressings.

- [Trader Joe's Organic Reduce Fat Coconut Milk 13.5 Fl Oz Each]
  A dairy-free alternative suitable for various recipes.

YOUR BODY DOES NOT HATE YOU, YOU'RE INFLAMED

- [Trader Joe's 21 Seasoning Salute (Pack of 2)]()**
  A salt-free blend of herbs and spices to enhance flavor without added sodium.

Beverages

Opt for drinks that are free from added sugars and offer health benefits.

- [Trader Joe's Organic Green Tea 20 Bags/box (pack Of 4)]
  Green tea is known for its antioxidant properties.

Shopping Tips

When selecting store-bought products:

- Read Labels Carefully: Avoid items with added sugars, refined oils, and artificial additives.

- Prioritize Whole Ingredients: Choose products where whole foods are the primary ingredients.

- Watch Sodium Levels: Opt for low-sodium versions to reduce inflammation risks.

- Choose Healthy Fats: Look for products containing sources of omega-3s and monounsaturated fats.

- Limit Added Sugars: Even natural sweeteners can contribute to inflammation if consumed in excess.

4-Week Meal Plan

Week 1

Monday

* Breakfast: Chia Pudding Power Bowl (p.43)
* Lunch: Mediterranean Chickpea Salad (p.55)
* Dinner: Coconut Turmeric Chicken Thighs (p.66)

Tuesday

* Breakfast: Green Smoothie with a Punch (p.44)
* Lunch: Thai-Inspired Rainbow Veggie Wraps (p.59)
* Dinner: Wild Salmon Bowl with Turmeric Quinoa (p.53)

Wednesday

* Breakfast: Golden Milk Oats (GF) (p.50)
* Lunch: Zucchini Noodles with Pesto & Grilled Chicken (p.56)
* Dinner: Eggplant & Lentil Curry (p.76)

Thursday

* Breakfast: Avocado & Smoked Salmon Toast (GF) (p.47)
* Lunch: Cauliflower & Chickpea Curry Bowl (p.60)
* Dinner: Grilled Chicken with Chimichurri & Roasted Veggies (p.80)

Friday

* Breakfast: Sweet Potato & Greens Hash (p.42)
* Lunch: Sardine & Avocado Salad Plate (p.58)
* Dinner: Moroccan-Spiced Chickpea & Spinach Stew (p.71)

Saturday

* Breakfast: Almond Flour Pancakes with Berry Compote (p.46)
* Lunch: Seared Tuna & Avocado Nori Rolls (p.61)

YOUR BODY DOES NOT HATE YOU, YOU'RE INFLAMED

* Dinner: Grass-Fed Lamb & Root Veggie Tagine (p.65)

Sunday

* Breakfast: Leftovers for Breakfast (Yes, Really) (p.51)
* Lunch: Roasted Veggie & Hummus Plate (p.62)
* Dinner: Bison & Veggie Skillet (p.77)

Week 2

Monday

* Breakfast: Turmeric Quinoa Porridge (p.45)
* Lunch: Wild Salmon Power Salad (p.100)
* Dinner: Slow Cooker Turmeric Chicken & Veggie Soup (p.75)

Tuesday

* Breakfast: Sautéed Veggie & Tofu Scramble (p.49)
* Lunch: Rainbow Slaw (p.101) + Miso-Glazed Cod with Broccoli & Shiitake (p.87)
* Dinner: Butternut Squash & Ginger Soup (p.91)

Wednesday

* Breakfast: Coconut Yogurt Parfait (p.48)
* Lunch: Curried Chickpea & Kale Crunch Salad (p.104)
* Dinner: Zucchini Lasagna (Grain & Dairy-Free) (p.72)

Thursday

* Breakfast: Chia Pudding Power Bowl (p.43)
* Lunch: Thai-Inspired Chicken Lettuce Wraps (p.83)
* Dinner: Hearty Sweet Potato & Kale Stew (p.93)

Friday

* Breakfast: Green Smoothie with a Punch (p.44)
* Lunch: Sardine & Olive Protein Salad (p.106)
* Dinner: Herb-Crusted Wild Salmon with Garlic Greens (p.64)

Saturday

* Breakfast: Almond Flour Pancakes with Berry Compote (p.46)
* Lunch: Warm Quinoa & Roasted Veggie Salad (p.102)

* Dinner: Stuffed Bell Peppers (Quinoa + Turkey) (p.79)

Sunday

* Breakfast: Golden Milk Oats (p.50)
* Lunch: Roasted Broccoli & Tahini Salad (p.107)
* Dinner: Mushroom & Wild Rice Soup (p.97)

Week 3

Monday

* Breakfast: Spiced Quinoa Porridge with Apple & Nuts (p.119)
* Lunch: Mediterranean Chickpea Salad (p.55)
* Dinner: Thai Coconut Curry Soup (p.94)

Tuesday

* Breakfast: Avocado & Smoked Salmon Toast (GF) (p.47)
* Lunch: Grilled Mackerel with Ginger Bok Choy (p.74)
* Dinner: Lentil & Sweet Potato Curry (p.54)

Wednesday

* Breakfast: Turmeric Quinoa Porridge (p.45)
* Lunch: Gut-Healing Fermented Veggie Salad (p.108)
* Dinner: Coconut Curry Shrimp & Veggies (p.78)

Thursday

* Breakfast: Coconut Yogurt Parfait (p.48)
* Lunch: Zucchini Noodles with Pesto & Grilled Chicken (p.56)
* Dinner: Moroccan Chickpea & Tomato Stew (p.96)

Friday

* Breakfast: Chia Pudding Power Bowl (p.43)
* Lunch: Avocado, Grapefruit & Arugula Salad with Honey-Mint Citrus Dressing (p.105)
* Dinner: Golden Turmeric Chicken Soup (p.89)

Saturday

YOUR BODY DOES NOT HATE YOU, YOU'RE INFLAMED

* Breakfast: Leftovers for Breakfast (p.51)
* Lunch: Cauliflower Tabbouleh with Wild Salmon (p.81)
* Dinner: Baked Trout with Lemon-Herb Quinoa (p.69)

Sunday

* Breakfast: Sautéed Veggie & Tofu Scramble (p.49)
* Lunch: Rainbow Slaw + Hummus Plate (p.101)
* Dinner: Spiced Lentil & Spinach Stew (p.90)

Week 4

Monday

* Breakfast: Almond Flour Pancakes with Berry Compote (p.46)
* Lunch: Seared Tuna & Avocado Nori Rolls (p.61)
* Dinner: Eggplant & Lentil Curry (p.76)

Tuesday

* Breakfast: Green Smoothie with a Punch (p.44)
* Lunch: Warm Quinoa & Roasted Veggie Salad (p.102)
* Dinner: Turkey Meatballs in Spicy Tomato Sauce (p.85)

Wednesday

* Breakfast: Golden Milk Chia Pudding (p.110)
* Lunch: Wild Salmon Bowl with Turmeric Quinoa (p.53)
* Dinner: Veggie-Stuffed Acorn Squash with Tahini Drizzle (p.67)

Thursday

* Breakfast: Sweet Potato & Greens Hash (p.42)
* Lunch: Roasted Veggie & Hummus Plate (p.62)
* Dinner: Hearty Veggie & White Bean Soup (p.84)

Friday

* Breakfast: Spiced Quinoa Porridge with Apple & Nuts (p.119)
* Lunch: Curried Chickpea & Kale Salad (p.104)
* Dinner: Miso-Glazed Cod with Broccoli & Shiitake Stir-Fry (p.87)

Saturday

* Breakfast: Chia Pudding Power Bowl (p.43)
* Lunch: Sardine & Avocado Salad Plate (p.58)
* Dinner: Bison & Veggie Skillet (p.77)

Sunday

* Breakfast: Coconut Yogurt Parfait (p.48)
* Lunch: Wild Salmon Power Salad (p.100)
* Dinner: Gut-Healing Bone Broth & Veggie Soup (p.95)

Recipe Index

YOUR BODY DOES NOT HATE YOU, YOU'RE INFLAMED

T

W

YOUR BODY DOES NOT HATE YOU, YOU'RE INFLAMED

Made in United States
Cleveland, OH
05 June 2025

17345810R00083